GLOW
FROM WITHIN

JOANNA VARGAS

WITH SARAH DURAND

HARPER WAVE

An Imprint of *HarperCollins*Publishers

GLOW

FROM WITHIN

CONTENTS

I'm going to make you a promise right now: in just a few short months, you can have the fabulous, radiant skin you've always wanted. It doesn't matter if you've suffered from acne since you were a teenager, if you're bothered by persistent dry or itchy spots on your cheeks, or if the fine lines around your eyes and mouth make you look older than you really are. Whatever your issues may be, you can achieve healthy, pliable, smooth skin that positively glows from within.

Here's the amazing secret no one else will tell you: the quality of your skin is not about your skin type, and it has nothing to do with how many expensive products you can afford. Great skin doesn't require undergoing harsh or invasive treatments that leave you looking sun-scorched. It's not just about just being blessed with good DNA, either; even if your seventy-year-old mother looks fifty, you won't necessarily march into middle age problem-free. To consistently achieve that clear, bright, moisturized look that so many celebrities enjoy, all that's required is a solid skincare routine.

That's right. Armed with a strong, reliable, and consistent plan of action, you can enjoy gorgeous, glowing skin *for the rest of your life.*

But what exactly does a great routine entail? Is having beautiful skin as easy as doing the same thing—with the same products—morning and night, day after day? Yes, mostly, but you also need to understand *why* you're doing it. You have to start with an understanding of the unique biology and structure of your skin, including how aging, nutrition, products, environmental factors, and genetics affect it. If you're not truly familiar with something, you can't fix it—and that goes for your skin as well as anything else in your life. This knowledge base about your nutrition, beauty, and self-care routines is the *only tool you need* to take your skin to the next level.

It's important to keep in mind that everyone's skin is unique, so what works for you might not be what works for your friend or your sister. For example, I recommend the moisturizing benefits of marula oil to many of my clients, but I break out within hours of applying it. It's just *not* the right ingredient for me. In this book, I won't lay out a one-size-fits-all approach for your routine. Instead, I'll show you which *five steps* are essential for everyone, what ingredients are the best for which skin types or conditions, why certain foods might benefit or harm your skin, and which procedures might be a good fit for your price point or particular issue. My goal is to arm you with both a solid education and practical tools, providing just enough room for you to experiment with your skincare routine in a smart—and fun—way!

But who am I to tell you how to treat your skin? There are dozens of beauty books out there, written by amazing dermatologists, makeup artists, bloggers, and cosmetic industry pioneers—all promising life-changing results. Why should you listen to me? The short answer is, because I'm an aesthetician—or facialist, as my job is commonly called—and I understand healthy skin and top-notch skincare products in a way most others don't. I spend my days getting up close and personal with skin in a very particular way. A dermatologist's job is to diagnose and fix a problem. My job is to both nurture your skin in the moment *and* help you create a long-term, sustainable skincare program. In addition, dermatologists often take an invasive approach—like injecting fillers and Botox—to solving cosmetic issues, while my interventions are gentle, ranging from dry brushing to exfoliation to light therapy. And unlike most makeup artists, I understand the ingredients that go into skincare products and cosmetics at the chemical level, and I help my clients choose the products that best support the needs of their skin. Now, I'm not trying to *sell* you products (though I do have a line of my own). I know that your skin type, budget, current product preferences, and specific skin concerns all play a role in what types of products you buy. My life's purpose is to help women understand the unique nature of their skin, create a plan to support it, put that plan into action, and then step back and watch as they start to look and feel more confident and beautiful than they have before.

I absolutely *love* what I do, but in a lot of ways it's a career I came to by accident. Growing up in suburban New Jersey, I was close to my family and had a strong circle of friends, but I was an introverted, studious, and artistic kid. I loved to paint and take photographs in the privacy of my room or my backyard. The way I chose to express myself was through beauty, and by the time I was four or five, I collected more perfumes, lip glosses, bubble baths, and bottles of nail polish than anyone I knew. I was a product junkie, and I found the perfect partner in crime in my beloved grandma, who let me apply as much cream and blue eye shadow to her face as I wanted. My mom's side of the family comes from Mexico and Puerto Rico, and Latin women are usually very sophisticated when it comes to beauty. My grandma was a case in point, and that's why she indulged me. She didn't even complain when I tried to put hot rollers in her hair!

I went to private school, studied hard and made good grades, then enrolled at the University of Chicago—by anyone's measure the kind of place that would produce a responsible, upwardly mobile young adult who'd get a good corporate job after college. But I followed my passions instead, picking women's studies and photography as my majors. During my senior year, I had to write a thesis, so I settled on a project about the portrayal of women in society and the media. I asked dozens of my friends, classmates, and favorite teachers if I could photograph them in whatever state they felt defined their standard of beauty. Much to my shock, most of these women showed up for their photo shoots dressed in their favorite clothes—but without a speck of makeup on. Their faces were naked, yet they *still* felt stunning. Right at that moment, a lightbulb went off in my head: *What you put on your face* isn't *what makes you feel beautiful. Women feel authentically gorgeous when they express what's inside them instead.*

I shoved this thought to the back of my mind, and it stayed there. After graduation, I moved back east to New York City. I wanted to become a fashion photographer, but after about a year I realized I just didn't have what it took for a job like that. I was still so quiet, and a career where you need to be "on" all the time didn't play to my strengths. I was happiest with people one-on-one—like I'd been with my grandma. Plus, I was still a beauty fanatic, collecting all the red lipsticks and fancy creams I could get my hands on. I decided to go to beauty school, thinking I'd become a makeup artist, and when I told my family, they were *horrified.* I'd always been a free-spirited artist, but this was beyond kooky! As far as they were concerned, people who graduated from the University of Chicago did *not* throw away their degree to play with makeup for the rest of their lives.

I did what my heart told me to do, though, and I enrolled Manhattan's Christine Valmy International School for Esthetics, Skin Care and Makeup. I quickly learned that beauty school is a lot different than most people imagine. You're not just learning about shades of eyeliner or how to apply foundation; you're also taking classes about bacteriology and learning about layers of skin and the muscles and bones of the face. It was there that I began to understand that good skin isn't just about what you slather on in the morning or the genetics you were born with. Your skin

introduction

reflects the many parts of who you are and how you live and view your life. Skin is a *complex living organ*—and I wanted to learn all about it.

I fell in love with the process of facials right away. I adored taking care of people, making them feel good about themselves. The individualized care really spoke to me; each person's face felt like a puzzle I couldn't wait to put together. Most of all, though, I loved how facials brought out the best, most authentic version of a woman: an image she had created herself and never covered up with colors or shadows that filtered out who she truly was. Facials stripped my clients down to their pure form, allowing me to bring out the beautiful person inside.

The problem with beauty school, though, is that it offers no clear plan for finding your own way within the industry. I didn't have a mentor at Christine Valmy, and my desire to learn more wasn't met with any obvious paths to follow. So I decided to give myself a year to work at an organic day spa in Tribeca, and then I planned to search for what else the industry had to offer.

I gained a lot of valuable experience and knowledge in that first job, but I left bothered by one thing: most facials consisted of painful extractions, a peel, a little moisturizer, and then you were on your way, your face so red and sore you couldn't go back to work. There had to be a better process, and I knew I'd find it. By the end of the year, I stuck with my plan and branched out, taking a position with a dermatologist. The doctor I worked for ran a salon in conjunction with his medical office. He'd send patients to me after laser treatments or medical-grade peels, and I did my best to help them recover, reducing their inflammation or redness with a cow placenta facial or a series of moisturizing masks. These patients showed dramatic signs of skin irritation after their treatments. Again, couldn't you achieve clear skin without a harsh peel? I *knew* there was a gentler, yet still effective, way to get great skin. I left after a year, got a job at a different spa, and tried as hard as I could to forge my own unique path.

All through those early years, one of my favorite places to go was the New London Pharmacy in Chelsea. On the surface, it looked like an old-style pharmacy, complete with a drug counter in the back staffed by a few straight-laced pharmacists in white lab coats. But when I walked the aisles, it became a different place. The shelves held a treasure trove of beauty brands you could find only in Europe: amber-colored serums in medicine droppers, with exotic French names; lavender- and honeysuckle-scented perfumes; and rich, sweet-smelling creams made from all-natural ingredients I'd never seen on a label in America, where every beauty product was chemically based. The rumor was that the owner traveled to Europe as often as she could and brought back these beautiful, lustrous serums, oils, soaps, hair and nail conditioners, and perfumes in her suitcase. How was that even possible? I couldn't figure out how anything smaller than a shipping container could have carried it all. I used to wander New London's aisles, translating the labels as best I could, touching, smelling, sampling, and buying more than I could afford. This place was heaven to me, and so different than any other store I'd found in New York.

In 2006, when my son was just one year old, I decided to open my own salon. At a time when many salons were investing in $20 million build-outs, my husband and I found a space in Midtown Manhattan that was a cozy 290 square feet. The wall separating the treatment room from the front desk was so thin, you had to whisper so people waiting for their facials wouldn't overhear you. Social media was in its infancy in those days, so I publicized myself by calling everyone I knew, offering them facials, and praying that they would like their treatments enough not only to come back but also to spread the word. Luckily, the strategy worked! Soon I was doing eight facials a day.

Though those early days were exhausting, I knew I was onto something. One side of skincare focused on filler, Botox, peels, and extractions, while the "hippie" side was all about aromatherapy, relaxation, and whether to use lavender or patchouli essential oils on your face (trust me, there are far better—and less smelly—oils to use). I stood somewhere in the middle, taking a natural approach that got *results*. There were no spas that offered technology like LED light treatments, but mine did. I also tried to make my space feel as safe, comfortable, and supportive as possible. When I gave facials, I laughed with my clients, and we talked about everything from their boyfriends to their careers. They left feeling lighter, prettier, and like they'd just had a confidence-boosting heart-to-heart with a friend. The bonus for their skin was that I used organic products—some of which I'd created myself.

That's right. I also became an inventor. I remembered all the hours I'd spent in the New London Pharmacy and knew there weren't any nontoxic but effective skincare lines in the US, so in 2011 I started my own. I found a cosmetic chemist—whom I still work with—as well as a factory that's the only certified organic skin- and hair-product manufacturer in this country. Right from the start, I considered my chemist my partner. I could tell him exactly the kind of benefits I envisioned and the specific ingredients I thought might work, and he'd create the product I wanted. My first invention, my Daily Serum, took a few years to perfect, but my patience was rewarded because it's now my bestselling product. Luckily, now I'm much faster and can whip up something new in only a few months. I'm always trying to keep up on the latest trends, research, and technology, and I'll describe many of those in detail in this book.

I now have two salons—one in LA and one in New York City—and I still do at least four facials a day. I see a lot of celebrities, but most of my clients are people just like you. They're women and men who want to feel confident, with a beauty that glows from within.

My job isn't *just* to make your skin look pretty. Nor is it merely to make it feel soft, moisturized, exfoliated, and fresh for the hour to hour and a half that you're in my salon. I'm interested in the long-term health of your skin, so I focus on much more than indulging you. Healthy skin is a lifetime commitment; I never try to patch up a skin problem with a quick product recommendation or dashed-off advice like "Drink plenty of water and get some rest." Instead, I'm always thinking about what happens under the hypodermis—in your digestive and lymphatic systems, with your psychological state, daily routine, and more. After all, the skin's health and overall appearance are a great way to tell what's going on with your body internally. Trouble on the outside of the body means trouble on the inside, and if your skin breaks out or is sensitive, red, dry, or irritated in any way, it's because something below the surface isn't working for you.

My job starts when I first look at your skin. When a client lies down on a soft, well-cushioned table in one of my salons, I ask that they close their eyes and try to relax. I wrap a soft towel around their head, gently remove their makeup, then gaze at their skin in its raw state. I study them for a minute or so, taking note of the size and cleanliness of their pores, whether they have sun damage, if they have dry spots or an overall problem with moisture level, how elastic the skin appears to be, and whether there are any sensitivities. I think about the general canvas of their face, and how it relates to who they are. Are they old or young? A sun worshipper or someone who takes great care to protect their skin? Do they have known allergies or food sensitivities?

Throughout a facial, I walk my client through the basics of their skincare needs, demystifying and breaking down the jargon about what leads to clean, clear, happy skin. That's what I plan to do in this book as well. So many people I meet don't understand why skin reacts to certain foods, how hydration affects the skin, why certain light frequencies can help or harm you, or how often you should cleanse, exfoliate, or apply sunscreen, yet all these factors can make a world of difference in the health and appearance of your skin. Most of all, they don't have a consistent routine that executes that knowledge. I want *Glow from Within* to change that. The advice on every page is grounded in the sci-

introduction

ence I've studied and lifestyle-based wisdom I've learned over the past few decades. Think of it as both an encyclopedia and a directive on natural, noninvasive skincare.

We'll begin with an overview of an essential five-step routine that anyone can follow. Then we'll dive into the four fundamentals of a great skincare lifestyle, accompanied by short, actionable strategies that will help you map out a program you can use for the rest of your life. This routine offers easy, uncomplicated solutions, as demonstrated by my client Jake Gyllenhaal. One of the things I love about Jake is that he's very comfortable with who he is. And while he doesn't have a difficult skincare routine, he takes the time each day to care for his handsome face. He uses sunscreen, a good cleanser, and an effective serum, with a facial thrown into the mix every once in a while. He's proof that you can keep it simple and still look great.

By the end of this book, I hope you will not only understand skin better—I hope you will also grow to love it as much as I do. I want you to gain confidence in yourself and your skin so that you can go out and face the world without spending time worrying about what you look like. Beautiful, glowing skin can be a reflection of a healthy, vibrant life, and that's what I want for *all* of you.

GLOW
FROM WITHIN

one

UP CLOSE
AND
PERSONAL

S top what you're doing and go take a look at yourself in a mirror. What do you notice? Do you see delicate, fine lines around your eyes, above your lips, and in the corners of your mouth? Do you spot red patches on your upper cheeks, with tiny capillaries winding their way just under the surface of your skin? Or do you see a complexion that's clear, smooth, and even, with a pillowy, well-hydrated softness? Whatever you notice, take it in, and please don't judge. Your skin is telling a story about *you*. It's signaling how old you are, what you eat, how much you've slept, whether you've been sick or injured, or how much time you've spent in the sun. It's reflecting whether you're happy, stressed, nurtured, or sad. Your skin is mirroring the multifaceted story of your life, with all its joy and tragedy. Since the day you came into this world, your skin has been working for *you*—protecting, fighting, filtering, regenerating, and more—performing arguably the most diverse and complicated set of tasks of any organ in the human body.

The skin is amazingly complex, and every day I learn something new and fascinating about it. But while everyone's skin is unique—reflecting their DNA, heritage, and the internal and external stressors they've faced over time—the way our skin functions is universal. Across cultures, continents, and races, skin has roughly the same makeup and biology. Absent environmental factors, all skin types also age about the same way. Your skin is a living, breathing powerhouse working at all hours of the day and night, and if you understand it, you can make changes and implement routines that will make it healthier and more radiant.

glow from within

get inside your skin

Have you ever heard of the integumentary system? Neither had I, until I started beauty school. Along with your hair and nails, your skin is part of this vital system that acts as your body's protective shield. Coming in at just about 20 square feet, the skin is your second-largest organ, just smaller than the interior lining of your small intestines. The skin makes up 12 to 15 percent of the average person's weight, and it's your body's fastest-growing organ, shedding 30,000 to 40,000 of its 19 million cells a day and replacing them with new ones. It's also a storehouse for components of the body's other systems, including nerves, blood vessels, and lymphatic tubes. There's so much going on in your skin that, if you put one inch of it under a microscope, you'd see about 650 sweat glands, 20 blood vessels, 60,000 pigment cells, and 1,000 nerve endings. *Whew!* That's a lot of activity for something that's about 4 millimeters at its thickest.* Your skin is busy and overtaxed, and it frequently takes a beating—so you need to treat it well! We'll get to what you can do for your skin in a minute. First, I want you to understand more about what your skin does for you.

*Your skin is thickest on the soles of your feet and thinnest on your eyelids.

just below the surface

The skin has three major layers: the thin top layer, called the epidermis; followed by the thicker, meatier dermis; and below that, the hypodermis, the thickest, fattiest layer. Together, these three layers protect the body from bacteria and pollutants in the environment, serve as a filter for toxins that can't be handled by the body's other organs, prevent the loss of water and nutrients, regulate temperature, and help you feel sensations like cold, pain, and pressure.

Since the **epidermis** is the layer that's visible, most people assume that it's the only part of the skin that facialists are concerned with. In truth, the epidermis constantly works in conjunction with the skin's other layers. On its own, though, it's the center of cell activity, where cells are both created and sloughed off at the end of their short lives. Skin cells are formed at the bottom of the epidermis, and in the beginning they're fat and square. Over the course of a few weeks to a month, they flatten out and move up to the stratum corneum—the top layer of the epidermis. When they're almost completely flat and packed on top of each other in about twenty-five to thirty layers, they come off manually through exfoliation or desquamation, which is the

glow from within

body's harmless and unnoticeable shedding process. Ever wonder where all the dust lying around your house comes from? A lot of it is dead skin cells that have simply fallen off during desquamation. That may sound impossible (and totally gross), but on average, the body sheds about 35,000 skin cells every hour.

But what *are* skin cells? There are several different types, including keratinocytes, melanocytes, Langerhans cells, Merkel cells, and inflammatory cells, but the ones you should be most concerned with are keratinocytes and melanocytes. Keratinocytes make up about 95 percent of the skin cells in the epidermis, and they produce a fibrous protein called keratin, which gives your skin structure and resilience. Keratin binds cells to one another, giving your skin cohesion.

A second major type of skin cell found in the epidermis is the melanocyte. Melanocytes are irregularly shaped, lie at the base of the epidermis, and produce and store a substance called melanin, which is the pigment responsible for the color of our skin. Believe it or not, no matter what color your skin is, you have around the same number of melanocytes as any other person in the world, dark or fair. But it's the amount of melanin these cells produce that dictates your skin color, and that's determined by your genetics. If you produce no melanin, you have albinism, and if you produce a large amount, you will be very dark skinned. Melanin absorbs harmful ultraviolet rays, so your body produces more of it when you're exposed to the sun. But if you've spent hours in the sun, haven't burned, and instead have developed what you might consider a "healthy" tan, that doesn't mean you haven't damaged your skin. Your melanin has worked as hard as it can to protect you, and a tan is a signal that it's overtaxed and that you *must* put on sunscreen to avoid more long-term harm.

The **dermis** lies just below the epidermis, and it averages about 2 millimeters in thickness. Once believed to be an inert area of the skin, we now understand how active it is, containing a vast network of structures that are essential to the functioning of your entire body, including sweat and oil glands, nerve endings, hair roots, and blood and lymph vessels. Many of these structures extend up through the epidermis, like hair follicles, which are attached to tiny muscles, but many lie below the surface and stay there, like nerve endings. The dermis also consists of fibrous connective tissue made up of proteins, which helps protect the body from stress and strain, gives the skin strength, and provides elasticity.

While the many different proteins within the dermis are essential to the functioning of the skin, the ones that aestheticians and dermatologists are primarily interested in are collagen and elastin. Elastin makes up the connective tissue. It's what allows your skin to stretch and then bounce back. The second major

glow from within

protein is collagen, which is the most abundant protein in the human body, found throughout our major organ systems. It's particularly important to the skin, essentially holding it together. As you age, collagen production declines, and that accounts for the saggy skin, hollow cheeks, and general reduction in healthy "puffiness" that you may see in a lot of older people.

Just below the dermis is the **hypodermis**, or the subcutaneous fat layer. If the name doesn't say it all, this is where the fat in your skin in housed. Not just that, but the hypodermis is where 50 percent of your entire body's fat is stored! This layer is also your temperature-control center, protecting your body from overheating or getting too cold, as well as providing the padding for your muscles and bones. As you age, this layer of fat diminishes, which contributes to hollowness and droopy skin. The hypodermis also contains a network of connective tissue that attaches the skin to the bones, essentially keeping your skin from falling off your body.

Finally, the hypodermis contains a number of different types of cells, including macrophages, which are important immune system cells that help fight germs and other foreign substances. Its most abundant cell type, however, is fat cells, which, in addition to doing all the things I mentioned above, release a substance called leptin. Leptin tells the brain when to signal your body to stop eating.

as your skin ages

Now that you understand the form and function of your skin, you may be wondering what happens to it over time. The truth is that as far as skin is concerned, there is no turning back the clock; aging skin is part of a natural process that's determined in part by genetics. But there are some things that will make your skin age faster than others, and throughout this book, I'll address treatments, ingredients, and dietary tips that will help you ease into the aging process rather than having it overtake you. First, though, let's try to understand the many changes that occur within your skin over time.

Aging starts in earnest in your mid-twenties. I know, I know—that sounds *so* early, but it's reality, and it's why I always urge young people to take skincare seriously, even if they still look and feel like teenagers. It is never too early to start following the routines I lay out in this book, to pay attention to what products work best for your skin, to wear sunscreen daily (even young kids and babies!), and to eat right. If you can afford one, don't be shy about scheduling a facial, too. Your aesthetician will help guide you into a skincare regime that you can tailor to your needs as the years pass.

glow from within

What exactly happens to your skin as you age? Just under the top layer of your skin, the dermis begins to lose thickness, and from your mid-twenties until your golden years, its width decreases by 20 to 80 percent. The production of collagen and elastin slows down as well—and much of your skin's existing supply starts to break down—resulting in reduced resiliency and fullness.

In the epidermis, the skin becomes dehydrated, leading to the formation of wrinkles. This water loss happens in part because hyaluronic acid, a naturally occurring substance in our skin that helps us retain moisture, decreases starting in our forties. Further, the fatty acids in the stratum corneum can't bind and hold water, causing even more dehydration.

Between ages thirty and eighty, the rate of skin cell turnover declines between 30 and 50 percent, meaning that we don't shed cells as rapidly. This leads to dull, rough, flaky, patchy, or dry skin. Other skin cells don't form as quickly, either, causing a slower immune response in the body. This may be connected with a higher incidence of skin lesions like those caused by some cancers in older people.

Older people often have discolored skin, with darker patches in some places, areas of redness in others, and patches of white elsewhere. Skin discoloration is a hallmark of the aging process, and it occurs because—no matter your skin tone—the colors that combine to create your skin tone are red, blue, yellow, and brown. The red and blue are from oxygenated and unoxygenated hemoglobin in red blood cells, the yellow is from carotenoids and flavins, and the brown is from melanin. As you age—and especially if you've spent any amount of time in the sun—the activity of melanocytes becomes more erratic, leading to some dark patches and some white. Melanin levels also decline 6 to 8 percent per decade after age thirty, which means that older skin is more sensitive to the sun. If the skin has a yellow hue, that's because of a decrease in pigment and a decline in capillary activity under the skin.

Throughout this book, we'll talk more about some of the bad habits that can accelerate the aging process, but for now, know that sun exposure causes a whopping 90 percent of premature aging, with cigarette smoking, alcohol use, and poor diet wreaking havoc on your skin as well. But with a good routine, you can counteract this, so read on!

● ● ●

glow from within

a word about skin types

Whether your skin is oily, dry, a combination of both, prone to breakouts, or constantly red and irritated, you've probably decided that your skin falls into a certain category. Most people I've met are convinced that their skin is one certain type—and no other—and while I'm not saying that's wrong, I do think there are some gray areas when it comes to determining your skin type.

First, though, how do you decide which category you fit into? What if your nose is always oily, but in the summer, your cheeks are, too? Does that make you oily, combination, or sometimes one and sometimes the other? The way to determine your skin type is to look at yourself closely in the mirror. Is your skin textured and shiny, like an orange peel? Do you have large pores all over your face? If so, you have oily skin. If you have no visible pores—or very small ones—on your face, you have dry skin. If only the pores on your nose are large, then your skin is combination.

You might be surprised to hear that I estimate that a full *85 percent* of my clients have sensitive skin. Many of them don't realize it, either! That sensitivity may reveal itself as breakouts, redness, rosacea, or dry, flaky skin. If you're unclear about whether you have sensitive skin, the way to test is to press firmly in a few spots on your cheek. If you notice redness when you lift your finger, then you definitely fall into the "sensitive" category. Another way to check is to look at the crease of your nose, next to the nostrils, or your upper cheeks. If you notice that small capillaries under the surface have burst, causing redness, then you have sensitive skin.

Many assume that skin sensitivity is reserved for fair skin, but that's not the case at all. In my experience, more melanin-rich, darker skin tones may not wrinkle as prominently or quickly (because the cells in their dermis are packed more tightly), but their skin is actually more sensitive than lighter skin tones. I also find that many people with olive tones or darker complexions don't use sunscreen as regularly as lighter-skinned people, which can lead to problems. On my first beach vacation with my husband—who is blessed with more melanin than I am—he refused to put on sunscreen. I argued my point, to no avail, but after he got a massive sunburn and melasma—a brown or grayish-brown blotch—on his face, he finally saw the wisdom of preventive skincare. The truth is, *everyone* needs sunscreen, because sun exposure causes dark tones to age prematurely just as quickly as it does lighter skin.

Early in my career, it was trendy to think of beauty treatments only in terms of skin types. Honestly, this always struck me as

glow from within

outdated because there are so many constants in terms of skin. We all have collagen, and as we age, we all need products that will help to plump it up a bit. Everything from the turmeric you add to your soup recipe to a microcurrent treatment at the spa to the hyaluronic acid or almond oil you find in your moisturizer can boost collagen production—regardless of your skin type. There are also so many cutting-edge, innovative spa treatments available that are good for you whether you're oily, dry, sensitive, or none of the above.

Beauty begins deep inside you, and my wish for you is that you stop thinking about only the surface of your skin. Down in the dermis and hypodermis, and all around you in your heart, mind, and soul, there so many approaches you can take to improve your skin—and your life. In these pages I'll help you choose the right products, the best foods, and the most beneficial self-care techniques for you. I'll recommend some of my favorite products, and I'll also lay out some small tweaks to your routine you can make when you have a flare-up—like a breakout or a period of dry, flaky skin. Like I said, I'm convinced that beautiful skin is possible for anyone, once they put into place a solid routine that encompasses all aspects of their life. There's a gorgeous, glowing you just waiting to be unleashed, and I can't wait to show you how.

two

YOUR

NUTRITION

ROUTINE

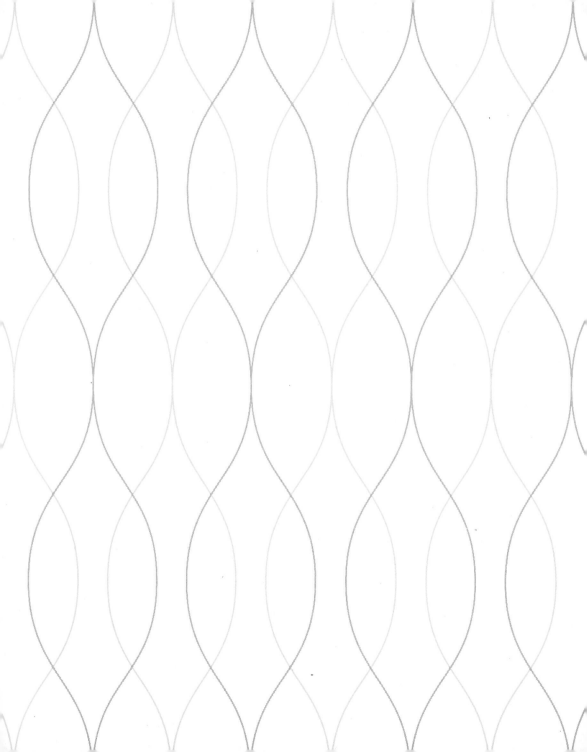

When I first became an aesthetician, the majority of women I saw were looking for a magic pill or treatment that would make their skin perfect in one session. Retin-A was all the rage for preventing and eliminating wrinkles; Botox was hailed as a savior for preserving your skin well into middle age; glycolic peels were so popular that I couldn't do a facial without discussing them or recommending products that contained glycolic acid.

But all these treatments have problems: Botox leaves your face frozen if it's overused, glycolic acid is too harsh for some people, and acids and retinols create sensitivity. Thankfully, in the two decades since

I began doing facials, our idea of skincare has evolved, and I don't think anyone is under the impression now that a gorgeous, glow-from-within complexion can be found under one lid or in one hour.

The most dramatic advancement I've seen in the beauty industry is our understanding of how what we put *into* our bodies affects our skin. Beauty isn't skin deep, and today most of my clients know that they need to eat nutritious meals, avoid particular foods, and drink enough water to achieve their own brand of agelessness. However, they often don't understand *why* and *how* these things affect their skin. They may have heard the advice that drinking too much alcohol dehydrates them, or that eating more vegetables will make their skin healthier, but they don't comprehend the mechanisms in their bodies that make this happen. That's why during every facial, I explain as carefully and clearly as possible how the body works so that my clients will come away with the knowledge of how their dietary and lifestyle choices affect their skin.

Every person is different, but there are some universal truths as far as establishing a great nutrition routine. Unlike other parts of this book, I won't order this section in terms of how your day proceeds, from morning to night. That's because some people like a protein-heavy breakfast, while others opt for a bowl of oatmeal, and some skip breakfast altogether. I'll focus on food categories instead, breaking them into what you should eat and what you should avoid. I'll also include a few quick tips and tricks I've learned over the years—easy, healthy choices you can implement in your day. This section will arm you with a knowledge of how nutrition impacts your bodily systems on the inside and ultimately your skin on the outside, allowing you to round out your routine with delicious, healthy foods that will make you feel and look better right away.

glow foods

GREENS

My number one nutritional beauty tip is absolutely my favorite skin fix: drink a green juice every day and try to eat green vegetables with every meal. Green smoothies are great, too, but I prefer fresh-pressed juices because when vegetable fiber is removed through the juicing process, your gut is able to absorb the nutrients more easily. Vegetables help keep your digestion healthy and provide tons of essential vitamins and minerals.

When absorbed, these nutrients help your body produce oxygen-rich blood cells. As the cells flow to the surface of your skin, your skin becomes oxygenated, giving you a fresh, dewy glow. Juicing is so great for your skin, in fact, that every single celebrity client I see follows this tip, and it shows all over their clear, clean, radiant complexions.

The skin relies heavily on the proper functioning of the lymphatic system, which is a network of vessels that carry a substance called lymph through your body and toward your heart. As part of the immune system, we have about six hundred lymph nodes in our bodies. These nodes swell because of infection, a buildup of white blood cells, or because of bacteria or toxic substances in the body. Lymph travels through the nodes, clearing them out, and it also helps our bodies absorb fats and fat-soluble substances, rids our tissues of liquids, and maintains the balance of fluids in our blood and tissues.

Unlike the vascular system, with the body's powerful heart at its center, our lymphatic system doesn't have its own pump. The only way lymph is able to move through the body is when it's squeezed through its vessels via the movement of our muscles. Think about how you look when you're sick or hungover or have eaten a few too many sugary foods. You look puffy and washed-out, like your body isn't in balance. Part of the reason that occurs is because your lymphatic system isn't draining your tissues as effectively as it should, struggling because of weakness and a lack of energy. What helps our muscles get stronger and allows them to move more easily and efficiently? Good nutrition. And *that's* what you can find in greens.

What kinds of greens should you be piling on your plate or drinking in your juices? First off, don't just limit yourself to vegetables—many fruits will give your skin a boost as well. Just bear in mind that many fruits are high in sugar, so I advise you to take in more vegetables than fruit and to look for low-GI fruits (those that have a lower effect on your blood sugar levels) like apples, strawberries, and kiwis. Some of my favorite green foods are kale, spinach, lettuce, celery, parsley, cucumber, and green apple because they not only taste delicious but are also chock-full of nutrients. Recently, pure celery juice—taken on an empty stomach—has been hailed as a superfood for its ability to clear skin, aid digestion, reverse chronic inflammatory and autoimmune conditions, boost energy, help with weight loss, and more. Celery juice contains vitamin C, folate, potassium, and vitamin A, so it's a nutrient-rich veggie that benefits everyone. While I don't drink it straight, some of my clients do, and they've seen dramatic results in their health and appearance. But I believe great things can happen with *any* green juice taken daily.

Here are some of the main vitamins and minerals you want to consume to keep your skin glowing:

- Vitamin C is found in large concentrations in the epidermis and dermis, so it's a natural component of skin that evens pigmentation, increases elasticity, brightens complexion, and improves skin's resilience. You can find it in citrus fruits, strawberries, broccoli, and spinach.

- Vitamin E is absorbed through nutrients and transported from the blood to the skin by sebum. It assists in absorbing the sun's harmful UV rays, calms inflammation, and helps to repair free radical damage. Vitamin E can also help combat dryness, even skin tone, and boost collagen. You can find it in avocados, bell peppers, mangoes, and kiwis, as well as in wheat germ oil and nuts, such as almonds and hazelnuts, and sunflower seeds.

- Vitamin D helps create new cells, which strengthen the immune system and prevent inflammation. This decreases the body's oil production, thus helping to prevent acne. Vitamin D is produced naturally when our bodies are exposed to sunlight—even when we're wearing sunscreen—but it can

glow from within

also be found in foods like eggs, fish, and fortified grains. Many people are deficient in this vitamin, so it's important to make sure you are getting enough of it, whether through diet or supplementation.

- **Vitamin K** This vitamin is present in kale, spinach, lettuce, and cabbage and helps promote blood clotting, which in turn eliminates stretch marks, spider veins, scars, and dark circles under your eyes.

- **Vitamin B$_2$** This vitamin is also known as riboflavin, and a deficiency of it has been proven to cause acne. Eating it in proper amounts (the recommended daily allowance is 1.3 milligrams for men and 1.1 milligrams for women) is essential for healthy skin, hair, and nails. It can be found in foods like green leafy vegetables, beans, and almonds.

- **Zinc** Duke University and the Department of Dermatology at SUNY Downstate Medical Center in New York have shown that this antioxidant can help reduce acne and boost the immune system. You can find zinc in red meat, legumes, asparagus, spinach, and almonds.

● ● ●

WHAT ARE FREE RADICALS?

Free radicals are molecules that have lost electrons and become unstable. Free radicals exist within cells, and they're formed when you are exposed to environmental stressors like sunlight or pollution or to viruses, parasites, fungi, or bacteria; or when you consume too much chemically altered fat, sugar, or alcohol. Free radicals attack DNA (your genetic material), protein receptors (proteins in the cell membrane that bind to external molecules), and enzymes (protein molecules that speed up chemical reactions in cells), and they destroy mitochondria (the energy plants of your cells). All this damage at the cellular level can pave the way for cancer and a host of other serious illnesses. As far as your skin's concerned, free radicals can wreak havoc on your collagen production, which leads to premature aging. Why would your body produce molecules that are so destructive? Because they also offer some benefit, including helping the immune system fight viruses, parasites, fungi, bacteria, and other nasty things that can invade your body.

FATS

Many people only worry about their fat consumption as it relates to their weight, cholesterol levels, and heart health. The fact is, though, that eating the right kinds of fat is essential to your well-being and the well-being of your skin. Each of your skin cells is surrounded by two layers of fat that make up the cell wall, and if you don't eat healthy dietary fats, those walls will weaken. This was confirmed by a study published in the *American Journal of Clinical Nutrition*, which concluded that women with a higher intake of healthy fats have fewer wrinkles and firmer skin tone—a result of strong skin cells.

But what exactly *are* healthy fats? They're not the trans fats found in french fries, doughnuts, potato chips, or other fried or processed snacks. The trans fats found in junk food are made with industrially produced vegetable oils that have had hydrogen added to make them solid. These fats are no good for your skin or the rest of you—consumption of trans fats has been linked to an increased rate of Alzheimer's, cancer, heart disease, obesity, and other diseases.

A good intake of healthy fats consists of a combination of omega-6 and omega-3 fatty acids—both of which are poly-unsaturated fats that can't be produced by the body—as well as omega-9 fats, a monosaturated fat the body does produce but that can also be obtained through foods. Omega-3 fats are found in oily fish like salmon, cod, tuna, halibut, mackerel, and sardines, as well as in walnuts, pumpkin, and dark green leafy vegetables like spinach and kale. In addition to helping with cell structure, omega-3s are anti-inflammatory, and they suppress insulin-like growth factor 1 (IGF-1), lessening red patches and acne. Omega-6 fats are found in corn oil, soybean oil, mayonnaise, sunflower seeds, pistachios, almonds, and more, and while we need to eat them in order to have energy, they can cause inflammation when the ratio of omega-3s to omega-6s is off. In addition to our bodies producing them, omega-9 fats are found in avocados, olive oil, and cashews, and they work to reduce cholesterol, inflammation, and triglyceride levels, as well as helping your epidermis retain moisture. Further, a study in the *American Journal of Clinical Nutrition* found that adding some avocado to a salad increased the absorption of vitamin E, beta-carotene, and lycopene fifteen times the average rates. These nutrients help protect your skin against sun damage from UV rays, and that, in turn, helps prevent the effects of aging and skin cancer.

The problem is that the average American diet consists of too many omega-6 acids and too few omega-3s and -9s. The recommended ratio of omega-6 to omega-3 is four to one, but most of us currently eat at least ten to one! So, in short, you can ensure you're getting a healthy amount of all the right kinds of fats by eating more oily fish and leafy green vegetables, as well as avoiding processed snacks, many of which are made with omega-6 oils. I also recommend adding avocados to your diet because they are good for your skin in so many ways. Your skin will thank you!

PROTEIN

The role protein plays in exercise is hardly ever overlooked—think of all the muscle-bound weight lifters you've seen guzzling down protein shakes—but it's often ignored when it comes to skincare. Trust me: protein is one of the most important elements to building strong, pliable, healthy skin.

Protein is a nutrient that's made up of amino acids, which are compounds within your cells. As one of the major building blocks of your body, protein makes up your muscles, skin, bones, and blood; it helps synthesize hormones and enzymes; and it keeps your immune system functioning at optimal levels. Without sufficient protein intake over time, your muscles begin to atrophy, your metabolism slows, and you may feel lethargic, struggle to lose weight, or start to lose your hair.

The typical American diet is heavily reliant on animal protein, so if you include eggs, milk, and meat in your diet, you're probably just fine. However, while animal protein contains all nine essential amino acids needed for optimal health, most plant proteins—except for soy—do not. Unfortunately, that's why many of my vegan clients suffer from skin problems in ways that my clients who eat animal protein do not. Their skin is less elastic than it should be for their age, and that makes them look drawn, stretched, and older than they are. This is not a slight against vegans; it's just an unfortunate result of not consuming certain proteins.

Let me give you an example: I have a beauty editor friend who is also a longtime client. I remember our first few appointments like they were yesterday. Even though she was only thirty, her skin's elasticity was more like that of someone in her sixties. Her face *looked* fine at first glance, but when I touched it, it moved, wiggled, and lifted like Jell-O. I was beyond alarmed! She was very pale, so the problem wasn't sun exposure. She didn't smoke, was very fit, and, in general, seemed like the picture of health. So what was it? Then it hit me: she had been following a vegan diet for about ten years. When I asked her how much protein she ate, she explained that while she knew she was supposed to be mindful of consuming enough, she often just lived on salad and vegetables, avoiding protein-rich foods like beans, nuts, and tofu. There it was. The body—everyone's body—needs protein to survive. Because her protein intake was so low, her body had tapped into her collagen and elastin reserves. I sent her to my go-to functional medicine doctor, Dr. Frank Lipman, to sort out a healing plan for her. The result? Stronger skin, a healthier complexion, and a great glow.

Remember, collagen and elastin are two components that make up your skin. Collagen provides your skin's structure, making it plump, fleshy, and strong, while elastin gives it stretch and the ability to bounce back when wrinkled up or pulled. Both substances are made up of protein, so it follows that if you're not getting the right kinds of amino acids in the right amounts, the levels of collagen and elastin in your skin will decrease.

If you avoid consuming animal protein, I recommend eating plenty of vegetarian proteins like tofu, tempeh, seitan, lentils, quinoa, nuts, and beans. Cutting out animal protein also tends to deprive you of zinc, a nutrient that's central to cell division and antioxidant activity. Not having enough zinc in your diet may lead to eczema and acne, and because zinc helps build up collagen, it reduces fine lines and wrinkles. You can find zinc in asparagus, spinach, almonds, pumpkin seeds, or any number of daily supplements.

You can't enter a juice bar without seeing row after row of protein powders, so many people assume that they can easily get their daily protein ration through supplementing. This is mostly true—but your skin may suffer for it. I'm a big fan of whey powder because it's so high in protein and the body breaks it down it very easily, but it's made from dairy, which gives some people trouble. It also intensifies the production of IGF-1 in the body. Insulin ups the amount of sebum your skin produces, and that increases the likelihood you'll develop acne. In addition, whey protein can trigger the production of androgens, hormones that increase oil production. Finally, many powders are highly processed, full of sugar, or—*gasp*—high in heavy metals like mercury. So if you rely on powders for your protein hit, be sure to read labels closely and choose a clean product.

If you do eat animal protein, I recommend steering clear of too much red meat, and filling up instead on fish like wild salmon and mackerel, which are full of omega-3 fatty acids (remember, getting enough fat is crucial for glowing skin!). Tuna, salmon, and shellfish like lobster and crabs are also full of selenium, which, along with vitamin E, helps keep your skin smooth and free of wrinkles.

● ● ●

glow from within

WATER

Your skin is composed of 30 percent water, so it figures that if you don't drink enough water, your skin will suffer, right? Yes, but the issue of dehydration and how it affects your skin is more complicated than you might think.

First off, dry skin is not the same as dehydrated skin. Dryness means you were born with fewer oil-producing glands, so your skin doesn't produce enough sebum. When you don't have enough oil in your skin, you don't have a strong protective barrier against environmental stressors, and your skin doesn't retain moisture as well as it should. That's why it may look dull, flaky, or rough.

Dehydration is a lack of water in your skin, not oil. Your skin can become dehydrated as a result of environmental stress (like not using a humidifier while you sleep in the cold, dry winter), improper use of products (like not using enough moisturizer) or using the wrong products (such as a drying soap), excessive caffeine or alcohol intake, or—you guessed it—not drinking enough water. Dehydrated skin can appear red, inflamed, or irritated and, when pinched, may not bounce back or may tent up in a wrinkly shape. It also may be oily or congested, because your skin produces excess oil to compensate for the lack of water. Because blood vessels constrict when the body doesn't have enough water, the skin may appear ashen, and you may have chapped lips and dark circles under your eyes. If your skin is rough and flaky, though, it's probably because of internal inflammation or, less likely, dryness—*not* because of dehydration.

Research on the effects of drinking water on your skin is somewhat limited, but one study, published in the *International Journal of Cosmetic Science*, compared images taken with a sonogram and concluded that adequate water intake improves the skin's thickness and density. The study also showed that proper hydration improves the skin's ability to retain water and helps prevent it from losing water. Hydrated skin cells swell, which makes the skin look plumper, thus reducing the appearance of fine lines and wrinkles. But does adequate hydration actually *reverse* the aging process? Not really. You need more than that. For example, if your skin is dehydrated, you should exfoliate to clear dead skin cells and make way for new cells that can retain moisture. You should use a heavier moisturizer—especially on top of a serum—and try products with hyaluronic acid, which helps your skin hold more moisture.

Obviously, drinking enough water is important for your overall health. But how much is "enough"? The old standard is that you should drink eight 8-ounce cups of water a day, but the truth is that the amount of water you need is based on your size, activity level, the temperature of the air, and what you eat. The National Academy of Medicine, European Food Safety Authority, and National Health and Medical Research Council of Australia have all published reports that recommend that men drink between 8.5 and 12.5 cups of noncaffeinated beverages a day, while women need somewhere between 7 and 9 cups. If you're pregnant or nursing, however, you need more.

How can you tell if you're dehydrated? First and foremost, if you feel thirsty, you're already 1 to 2 percent dehydrated. The second marker is your weight. Your baseline weight can be determined by getting on the scale at the same time each day and finding three similar weights. The median is your baseline weight, and being one pound under it means you're one pint of water dehydrated. A third way to tell is by your urine. If you go to the bathroom and see that your urine is straw colored or light yellow, you're not dehydrated. If it's clear, you're overhydrated, and if it's brown, you're retaining water and need to hydrate as soon as possible. Finally, if you work out and don't sweat, you need to drink more water. If you're dehydrated, the body can't pump blood *and* sweat, so it will skimp on the latter for the sake of the former.

Just bear in mind that it's unrealistic to expect that you'll never be thirsty or always have perfectly straw-colored urine. Hydration levels fluctuate, and it's the average that's most important—for your health and your beautiful skin!

HERBS AND SPICES

One of my favorite cooking strategies is to add fresh herbs and spices to meals and beverages. It's such an easy way not only to punch up the flavor of any dish but also to improve your skin. While no one herb or spice can act as a magic bullet to erase your wrinkles or stubborn acne, the herbs and spices listed here have proven anti-inflammatory and antioxidant properties that promote skin health. Less than a teaspoon a day of any of them can make a real difference.

- **Turmeric** This bright orange, slightly pungent spice contains a chemical component called curcumin that's a great antioxidant. Antioxidants are molecules that are famous for fighting the damaging effects of free radicals, and curcumin is especially effective when it comes to combatting sun damage. (For more information on antioxidants, see pages 86 and 90.) Curcumin is also anti-inflammatory, so it helps prevent the breakdown of collagen. A lot of people add turmeric to their soups and stews to give an earthier, more peppery flavor, but you can also take it in supplement form.

- **Rosemary** This terrific little herb increases the elasticity of your skin and has anti-inflammatory qualities, which will help your skin look less puffy and reactive. Rosemary is loaded with iron, calcium, and phytonutrients, which help prevent damage from free radicals, especially those due to exposure from the sun. Many people love steeping rosemary in tea, but you can also add it to soups, stews, meats, and vegetables.

- **Ginger** This root is absolutely loaded with antioxidants. It improves your skin's elasticity and evens out its tone, and if you apply it topically a few times a day on scars that are lighter than the surrounding skin, you'll notice how dramatically your skin tone blends together in only a few weeks. I love steeping ginger into a tea with a little honey and lemon; it's soothing for the stomach and smells absolutely divine.

- **Cinnamon** This delicious, aromatic herb isn't just for cakes and cookies! Cinnamon is loaded with antioxidants. It also slows down glycation—the process that binds sugar and protein in our bodies, which can break down collagen and elastin—so it promotes plumper, more pliable skin.

● **Fennel** With a licoricelike taste, fennel isn't for everyone, but it can do wonders for your skin if mixed with food or applied topically. It helps decrease your skin's redness and irritation, and the sensitivity that comes from too much time in the sun. A 2000 study published in the journal *Oncogene* also showed that anethole, the compound that gives fennel its smell and flavor, can block inflammation and carcinogenesis, the onset of cancer.

● **Cilantro** Like fennel, not everyone loves the taste of cilantro, but it too is a powerful antioxidant. It's also full of vitamin C, which increases its potency in fighting damage from free radicals. This helps lessen the appearance of wrinkles, sunspots, and uneven tone. Some of the chemical compounds in cilantro also bind with heavy metals in your system, so it can be a powerful detoxing agent against things like mercury, cadmium, and aluminum.

GUT HEALTH FOR GLOWING SKIN

You've probably heard some of the buzz about the importance of gut health. But what actually qualifies as a "healthy gut," and what does the state of your gut have to do with the state of your skin?

In a word, everything.

What is commonly referred to as the "gut" is really your gastrointestinal tract. Residing within your gut are approximately four hundred strains of bacteria that perform a variety of functions, including supporting digestion, the absorption of vitamins and minerals, and your immune system. This community of bacteria is collectively known as your microbiome.

Probiotics are live bacteria and yeasts that occur naturally in foods like yogurt and kefir as well as other fermented products like sauerkraut, apple cider vinegar, pickles, kombucha, miso, and kimchi. They also come in supplement form. Probiotics promote gut health because they help to keep a balance of good bacteria in the gut (preventing "bad" bacteria from crowding out the good kind), and those beneficial bacteria can then help your body absorb the nutrients it needs. A healthy population of good bacteria also helps the gut wall function properly, which can prevent leaky gut syndrome and autoimmune issues, all of which generate significant inflammation in the body.

I've seen great results when people add probiotics to their diet: acne can clear up in as little as two weeks, rosacea symptoms lessen, and skin tends to develop a generally rosier, more glowing appearance. A 2010 study in *Nutrition* looked at fifty-six people who suffered from acne and found that drinking a probiotic dairy drink every day for twelve weeks significantly cleared up their acne. And an Italian study concluded much the same: people who took a probiotic supplement in addition to their standard acne or rosacea treatment saw greater improvement than subjects who didn't take the probiotic supplement.

I have a celebrity client who, like many of my clients, gets photographed a lot. In the weeks leading up to the Met Gala, her skin broke out all around her mouth, especially right in the corners. I'm not a nutritionist, but I could tell she had candida, a fungal overgrowth caused by yeast in the gut. Because the gala was in two weeks, she didn't have enough time to see a nutritionist and change her diet, so I recommended a good probiotic and lots of LED light therapy. Within the first week, the one-two punch of probiotics plus light completely cleared up her skin and brought her inner glow back. The probiotic helped her digestive system function better.

What kinds of probiotics should you take, and how much? I recommend *Lactobacillus* and *Bifidobacterium* strains, specifically *Lactobacillus acidophilus*, *Lactobacillus plantarum*, and *Bifidobacterium longum*. Doctors recommend taking different amounts of probiotics per day, though it's generally assumed that between 300 million and 1 billion CFU (colony-forming units) is just fine. If you have a particular digestive issue like colitis or Crohn's disease, be sure to talk to your doctor before choosing a probiotic.

Recently, topical probiotics have become incredibly popular and are used widely in products like masks, serums, creams, mists, and more. This might sound crazy, but it makes sense: like our gut, the skin has its own biome, which consists of healthy bacteria that protect our skin and allow it to do its job (i.e., retaining moisture, protecting us from environmental stress, and shielding us from germs). Overcleansing, exfoliating, and the daily bombardment of toxins in our environment have stripped away some of this biome layer. Enter probiotic-infused products, which replenish this protective barrier with live microorganisms, prebiotics (which provide nourishment for existing skin bacteria), and postbiotics, the chemical by-products of good bacteria. I'm a big fan of these products. My clients have come away with less acne, diminished fine lines, less rosacea, improvements in eczema, and an overall healthy glow-from-within look. So, by all means, I recommend choosing products that contain prebiotics, probiotics, or postbiotics. One of my favorites is Solluna Feel Good SBO Probiotics+, which was created by my dear friend Kimberly Snyder (her book *The Beauty Detox Solution* is required reading for my team!).

moderation foods

DAIRY

In my experience, everyone's body reacts differently to dairy. Some of my clients break out at the sight of a glass of milk, while others can eat cheese all day and still look gorgeous. My advice when it comes to eating dairy is simply to pay close attention to how you feel (and how your skin looks) after consuming it. Only 10 percent of the population is truly lactose intolerant, or unable to digest lactose, the sugar that's one of the main components of milk. The achy stomach, diarrhea, bloating, respiratory problems, fatigue, joint pain, rashes, and acne that many people experience is often due to a sensitivity to casein—a protein found in dairy—rather than lactose intolerance. For these people, casein triggers an immune reaction during which white blood cells rush toward the perceived invader, causing inflammation.

Another point to consider if you're thinking about cutting back on or eliminating dairy is that nonorganic, pasteurized milk contains about sixty hormones. Many of these are the natural substances produced when a cow is pregnant or nursing—like progesterone and estrogen—but others are synthetic growth

glow from within

hormones used to increase a cow's milk production. These hormones are foreign to your body and may be associated with an elevated cancer risk. Drinking cow's milk also causes the body to increase its own production of male hormones, specifically testosterone and androgens. These substances—and in particular, the hormone called IGF-1—can lead to inflammation. Inflammation may then cause your skin glands and hair follicles to increase their oil production, in turn causing acne. In fact, a 2015 study found that the hormones in cow's milk increase skin's oil production by up to 60 percent. Further, one of the telltale signs of a dairy sensitivity is pimples around your chin and jawline. Breakouts in these areas are caused by a fluctuation in hormones—either those you create or those you ingest.

When new clients come to my salon, sometimes I can tell just by looking at them that they have a sensitivity to dairy. An actress client of mine was perplexed that her skin would only break out when she was working on a movie. Her skin looked great at home, no matter what time of year, but the second she started working on a film, she would break out in red patchy spots, with cystic acne along her jaw. We talked about the foundation she used during the shoots, and it was the same brand she wore at home. I told her to make sure the makeup artists cleaned their brushes every day, but they confirmed that they did so without fail. Could the problem be what she ate? Maybe, but her diet was impeccable. We kept talking and searching, and finally, we solved the mystery: my client drank several cappuccinos a day when she was on set, something she didn't do at home. Milk was the problem—her body just hated it. As soon as she cut out the cappuccinos, her skin cleared up!

Another reason why some people react to conventional dairy is that most dairy products available in the United States are made from homogenized milk. Homogenization is the industrial process of breaking down the fat molecules in milk so that a thick layer of cream doesn't develop at the top. This is convenient for many of us, but homogenization creates fats that our digestive systems aren't used to. If your system can't digest these fats, your gut may become inflamed, which results in greater oil production and more acne breakouts. Some people who have a bad reaction to conventional dairy products can tolerate raw milk and raw-milk products, which are not homogenized.

As I said, you may be someone who can eat dairy without issues. But if you have frequent breakouts—particularly around your chin and jawline—it's worth phasing dairy out of your diet, at least temporarily. Try to eliminate it for two weeks (it takes our bodies seven to ten days to filter out ingested hormones). If your skin starts to clear up in that time period, you may have found the cause of your breakouts. If you don't notice an improvement in your skin after two weeks, then you can reintroduce dairy.

Finally, if you do eat dairy, I encourage you to consume full-fat rather than low-fat because it contains more beneficial fats and protein; low-fat dairy is also often full of added sugar. And when you can, always try to look for pasture-raised, grass-fed, organic milk products.

GRAINS

Another popular diet trend is going gluten-free or grain-free, and many of my celebrity clients follow nutritional programs that eliminate grains and gluten. As with dairy, I've found that people's tolerance for grains is highly individual, and only a small portion of the population is truly allergic or intolerant. That said, grains, like dairy, do trigger an inflammatory response in the body. So when it comes to the appearance of your skin, I believe grains are best consumed in moderation. And if you are getting ready for a big event at which you'll be photographed, like a wedding, you may want to forgo grains for at least a week in advance to avoid any facial swelling or puffiness that can result from inflammation.

PLANTS DO A
BODY GOOD

Some of my clients who have a sensitivity to dairy worry about getting adequate calcium if they forgo milk. After all, it is recommended that women between nineteen and fifty years old consume 1,000 milligrams of calcium a day for bone health, and 1,200 milligrams for women fifty-one and older. Here's the good news: this essential mineral can be found in a number of nondairy foods. Here are a few of the top plant-based sources of calcium:

- Artichokes
- Barley
- Beans (pinto beans, black beans, and lentils)
- Broccoli
- Firm tofu
- Leafy greens (like mustard greens, kale, collard greens, and bok choy)
- Oranges
- Nuts (pistachios, walnuts, Brazil nuts, pecans, and peanuts)
- Rhubarb
- Sesame seeds

If you do choose to eat grains, I recommend sticking primarily with whole grains, rather than refined or processed grains. A whole grain contains fiber, which helps to slow digestion and thus your body's release of insulin, the hormone that's responsible for regulating blood glucose levels. Processed grains, which are found in cereals, crackers, bars, and other snack foods, are refined so they can last longer on supermarket shelves. These types of grains contain little to no fiber and are quickly digested and converted into sugar, and that's where your skin problems start.

In response to the elevated sugar levels in your gut, your body releases more insulin—which, in turn, causes inflammation. Inflammation then leads to redness, rosacea, puffiness, and an increase in oil production that can help acne develop. As refined grains break down, they also release IGF-1, which promotes an overproduction of skin cells called keratinocytes. This rapid multiplication is often associated with acne. Additionally, refined grains raise the levels of dehydroepiandrosterone (DHEA) and testosterone in your bloodstream. These two androgens are male hormones that stimulate the production of sebum in your skin, which can lead to acne and breakouts.

If you don't have any digestive issues with grains, my best beauty advice is to enjoy them in small amounts, and go for organic whole grains or sprouted grains (which contain niacin, B_6, and folate, which can help promote healthy skin) whenever possible.

CAFFEINE

If you're like most of my clients and friends, chances are the first thing you do when you get out of bed in the morning is pour a hot, steaming, delicious, desperately needed cup of coffee—or two. *Ahhh, now you can face the day.* I'm right there with you! I have no idea how I'd make it out the door—much less through the day—without a caffeine boost.

Let's start with the good news: caffeine is not necessarily bad for your skin. I say *not necessarily,* because if you drink caffeinated beverages to the exclusion of all others, you will have very dry, cracked skin and massive dark circles under your eyes. Caffeine is a diuretic in the same way that alcohol is, and if you don't do something to combat this, your skin will suffer. I recommend that in addition to the eight or so cups of water a day you should be drinking, you should have two cups of water for every one caffeinated beverage. Avoid sugary caffeinated drinks (as noted on page 53, sugar is no friend to your skin!) and consider swapping

glow from within

your coffee for green tea. It's a better choice because it reduces inflammation and acts as a powerful antioxidant, which helps you fight free-radical damage.

Coffee may actually be beneficial for some skin conditions, like rosacea, a condition characterized by patchy, pimply redness found most often on the cheeks and chin. Brown University's Department of Dermatology released a report in the *Journal of the American Medical Association* that found that women who drink four or more cups of coffee a day have a lower risk of developing the red, pimply bumps that characterize rosacea. Interestingly, the study found this benefit was uniquely connected to coffee— not other caffeinated beverages. Coffee may help you avoid developing skin cancer, too. According to a study published in the *Journal of the American Cancer Institute*, drinking four cups of coffee a day may reduce the risk of malignant melanoma by a whopping 20 percent! I'm not suggesting you regularly down ten cups of coffee a day, though. Caffeine can have lots of other unpleasant side effects, like stomach upset and increased levels of anxiety. But this research does suggest that drinking coffee may be beneficial for your skin.

Finally, a 2013 study showed that when applied topically, caffeine can work wonders on your skin. Rich in antioxidants, it helps lessen the fat accumulation in cells and increases blood flow. Coffee grounds are a terrific exfoliant, too, and I love mixing organic coffee into a scrub.

foods that dim your glow

ALCOHOL

Don't worry, I'm not going to suggest you stop drinking alcohol in order to have great skin. A lot of people love having a glass or two of wine with friends, and I think it's unrealistic to expect people to live 100% perfect, healthy lives—or to give up something they enjoy doing socially—in order to look good.

But "alcohol skin" is a real thing. I had a client who was going through a bad divorce and had been drinking hard for a few years. She took good care of herself otherwise—getting facials regularly and going to the gym—but the first time she came to me, I noticed something was wrong. Even though at age fifty, she appeared to have generally youthful skin, the moment she lay down on her back, the skin on her face sagged all the way back to her ears, with next to no elasticity. I also noticed that she had red, sensitized cheeks and bags under her eyes. I knew the culprit was alcohol.

Alcohol can affect your skin in significant ways, causing puffiness, dullness, dryness, and bags or dark circles under your eyes. Why does this happen? First and foremost, alcohol is a hepatotoxin, a chemical substance that damages the liver. One of the liver's main functions is to detoxify the blood, and alcohol interferes with that, meaning healthy skin cells can't regenerate properly if you've downed one too many drinks.

Alcohol also interferes with your body's absorption of vitamins, minerals, and antioxidants, including vitamins B, A, C, and D, calcium, zinc, iron, magnesium, selenium, tyrosine, and folic acid. Further, it flushes these essential substances out, leaving your skin susceptible to the free radicals created by environmental damage. When alcohol breaks down in your body, it releases toxins, and as your immune system responds to these toxins, it generates—you guessed it—inflammation. Your blood vessels also expand, which causes fluctuating blood pressure levels, leading to redness and rosacea. This finding is backed up by a 2017 study published in the *Journal of the American Academy of Dermatology*, which discovered, interestingly, that white wine and hard liquor had greater detrimental effects on women's skin than other types of alcohol.

Alcohol dehydrates you in two ways. First, it's a diuretic, so you go to the bathroom more when you drink. Second, it interferes with your body's production of vasopressin, a hormone that helps you absorb water. Basically, even if you *are* drinking water on a big, boozy night out, you are still likely to become dehydrated! And when you don't have proper moisture levels in your skin, you get dry patches or dull, lifeless skin.

What's a person to do if they drink too much one night, or drink regularly? The easiest thing you can do is to drink water to rehydrate. Because alcohol is very acidic, try sparkling water, which is alkaline, to help balance your pH levels. Second, eat green vegetables or drink a green juice to put the essential vitamins and minerals you've lost back into your body. You should also wash your face with a gentle cleanser that won't strip it of moisture. I like cleansers that contain vitamin C because it helps you fight damage from free radicals, and I am a big believer in the magic of charcoal for its detoxing properties (in fact, I make a charcoal soap called the Miracle Bar). Charcoal holds one thousand times its weight in toxins, which makes it perfect to help detox the skin and balance out acidic skin. After cleansing, spritz your face with rose water, which helps your skin to retain moisture. Follow with a terrific moisturizer or mask, especially one that contains hyaluronic acid, 1 gram of which can hold as much as 6 liters of water.

SUGAR

Today there is a growing public awareness that most of us eat too much sugar. In fact, it's estimated that one-third of the average American's diet is made of some form of sugar. One-third! Excess sugar consumption has been linked to any number of serious health issues, including diabetes, cancer, neurological diseases, and cognitive decline. It also damages your skin.

Sugar molecules bond with the protein and fat molecules in your body in a process called glycation. Glycation leads to the formation of substances called advanced glycation end products (AGEs) that accumulate in collagen. When they do, they begin interfering with the proteins and amino acids responsible for collagen production. As you know, collagen is the protein that makes up and maintains the structure of your skin, and when it breaks down, your skin begins to sag, wrinkle, wither, and look dull.

Sugar also raises your level of insulin—the hormone responsible for regulating glucose levels in your blood—leading to inflammation, especially in your digestive system. What does inflammation look like? Redness. When you have too much insulin in your body, your face becomes red, puffy, and irritated, either with rosacea's distinctive spider-webbing of burst capillaries or without it. Sugar also interferes with the binding of water molecules in your skin, which causes dehydration. To compensate, your skin will begin producing excess sebum, leading to breakouts.

If you've ever had a reddish or orangish, pimply, waxy rash around your lips and at the corners of your mouth, you may have assumed you were having an acne breakout. You were wrong. This unsightly condition is called perioral dermatitis, and it's caused by an overgrowth of bacterial yeast. Where does this come from? Sugar—either from the foods you eat or the booze you've been drinking. Try cutting out processed sugars and carbs for a few days to see if these symptoms disappear. Don't try to treat it with acne products; they won't work because it's not acne.

Sugar also causes your lymphatic system to slow down. The lymphatic system transports white blood cells and clears your body of cellular waste and debris. When it's impaired, bacteria and toxins aren't cleared out and healthy skin cells aren't replaced, so your pores become clogged, which can lead to breakouts. Finally, excess sugar in your bloodstream stimulates testosterone production, which leads to bigger pores and increased oil production. That means more blackheads, more pimples, and oilier skin.

The obvious way to prevent what some people call "sugar face" (red, pimply cheeks or saggy, lifeless, thin skin; fine lines; and dark circles under the eyes) is to avoid processed sugar altogether. That means no more cookies, cakes, or sodas, but it also means skipping pasta and pizza. Bread is made from white flour, and white flour is essentially a processed sugar. Most people who have bad acne or rosacea due to overconsumption of sugar will have clearer, healthier skin within a week of reducing their intake. Those with subtler problems—like fine lines, dark circles, or sallow skin—will start to glow brighter in three to four weeks. If you'd like to cut out even more sugar, take a look at the fruits you eat. Those that are higher on the glycemic index include pineapple, watermelon, and mango. Eating these fruits results in a sharper insulin spike than eating low-glycemic fruits like apples, oranges, and berries, so try eliminating high-sugar fruits first.

Another way to prevent the effects of sugar on your skin is to use skincare products that contain antioxidants like vitamin C, which help to combat the damage caused by decreased collagen and cell turnover. Vitamins B_1 and B_6—available by either taking over-the-counter supplements or eating foods in which they occur naturally—will also counteract some of the effects of AGEs, and drinking plenty of water will help you flush out some of the toxins that don't clear when your lymphatic system is compromised. Detoxifying teas like ginger, dandelion root, and green tea are also helpful.

three

YOUR SKINCARE ROUTINE

s far as your skin is concerned, what you put *on* your body is just as important as what you put *in* your body. With proper cleansing, sufficient hydration, gentle exfoliation, and a few more easy steps, everyone can see dramatic results in their skin in a matter of weeks. While it's important to think of the ingredients you apply to your face as nutrition—they should be organic, nonirritating, and, like a healthy meal, leave you feeling better than you did before—the products themselves aren't the full equation. Following a solid skincare routine day after day lays the foundation for healthy skin. Once you get into the swing of your own customized routine, it will become a habit like any other—one that you can keep for the rest of your life.

I believe there's a proper order your beauty routine should follow, so I'm going to share the five basic steps that most people (with a few small, skin type–specific exceptions) should follow at home every day. These simple actions don't take up a lot of time and won't break your budget, and they'll offer you plenty of freedom to choose the products and ingredients you want to use.

While I encourage you to stick with a routine, I also recognize that we're only human. There will be times when you're on an overnight flight and realize you forgot to bring your favorite cleanser, or nights when you party so hard that you crash into bed, fully clothed, without washing your face. It's okay. You can pick up where you left off the next day, and chances are high that your skin won't suffer for the lapse. And if your routine does go off the rails so badly that you break out; develop mean, dark circles under your eyes; or come down with the worst case of eczema you've had in your life, I've provided some simple tips for troubleshooting these acute situations in chapter 6.

There's a lot of information out there about products. Sorting through the hundreds of recommendations you find in magazines and blogs can be dizzying. I've been creating my own products for almost a decade, and I still find some of the difficult-to-pronounce ingredients to be beyond my comprehension! (I mean, what the heck *is* galactoarabinan?*) While I can't dissect every single ingredient you might find on a label, I will offer some insight into key terms you should look for. Hopefully you will come away from this chapter armed with the most vital information you need to make good choices—you'll understand what an acid is, how retinol works, and when and how to use a toner (if at all!).

Setting up a great skincare routine starts with the fundamentals, so we'll begin by looking at the treatments, techniques, and ingredients you'll need to get going. And while I'll recommend some of my favorite products on the market, please know that I recognize that everyone's needs and budgets are different, and you can still get amazing skincare without stretching beyond your comfort zone. Just choose wisely, and above all, pick products that fit your skin's needs and your lifestyle.

●　●　●

*In case you're wondering, it's an ingredient derived from the larch tree that speeds cell turnover for more youthful, vibrant skin. I use it in my Daily Hydrating Cream, and it is absolute heaven!

the five-step daily routine

step 1 ● CLEANSE

Cleaning your face sounds like the most basic thing in the world, but you'd be surprised by how many people get it wrong—or, worse, don't do it at all. Along with sun protection and moisturizing, gentle cleansing is one of the most important things you can do for your skin. In fact, it's so nice, you should do it twice.

Wait, what? Twice? That's right—removing your makeup is phase one of cleansing, while a good wash is phase two. The first removes surface debris, and the second cleans your pores. And if you don't do both steps, or you do them improperly, your skin will look dull, congested, or—depending on your skin type—overly dry or oily.

Proper cleansing is essential because it removes the oil, dirt, and environmental pollutants that build up on your skin every day. Many people with oily skin choose to wash in the morning and at night, but my skin tends to be on the dry side, so I only wash in the evening. If you have skin like mine, washing once a day is completely fine. But never, ever skip nighttime cleansing. If you fall into bed with your makeup on and sleep in it overnight, your skin cells won't be able to rejuvenate, and you'll very quickly lose luminosity; if you have oily skin, you'll break out. If you don't wear makeup and skip washing at night, your skin will still be covered in environmental impurities, and in the morning, any products you put on won't be able to penetrate through them—all that expensive moisturizer you slather on your face will accomplish nothing!

There are more types and brands of cleansers on the market than any intelligent person can wrap their brain around, so whatever you do, just remember to never use a cleanser that contains sulfate and never use over-the-counter bath or facial soap. Both contain industrial surfactants that can damage the skin. If you have dry skin and insist on using soap, though, seek out something with a natural foaming agent like sugar beets or coconut; these won't dry out your skin. Finally, avoid products that contain alcohol—it's not only unnecessary, it's also dehydrating if you have dry skin.

I'll start by describing makeup remover, then move into a few basic types of cleansers. You can choose whatever is best for you, but, like I said before, never skip the first step of removing your makeup. It's essential for clean, glowing skin.

•   •   •

makeup remover

I can't say it enough: you should always remove your makeup before you wash your face. I know, I know—adding an extra step seems like a lot of work, and I even groan about it sometimes. But trust me, it removes the junk on your epidermis and paves the way for a clear palette when it comes time to wash your face. I love micellar water because it contains fatty acids, which soothe the skin, and esters, which help strengthen the skin. You can also look for micellar water with cucumber, which soothes the skin, and vitamin E, which protects. Makeup removers that contain calendula flower extract, which cleans well and is calming for the skin, are also terrific. Coconut oil and jojoba oil may also work as makeup removers. They're both detoxing and chock-full of omega-3 fatty acids, and if you massage them into your skin using your fingertips, they'll clear away all your makeup.

cleanser • take your pick

1. **Foaming cleansers** are light and water-based; to use one, simply rub it onto your face in a circular motion, paying special attention to your hairline and jawline. If you've been

wearing a ton of thick, heavy makeup, you can try a foaming cleanser that contains an exfoliant. The scrubbing properties will ensure that you remove all the residue that your makeup remover may have missed.

2. **Oil-based cleansers** have become especially popular lately. In contrast to conventional wisdom, they're actually good for oily skin. They're soothing and anti-inflammatory, while also completely removing makeup and environmental build-up. Avoid petroleum-based cleansers, which will clog pores. Hazelnut oil and castor oil are terrific cleansers, as are olive oil (which is an anti-inflammatory skin softener) and grape seed oil (which contains soothing antioxidants). If you have oily skin and don't want to cleanse with an oil, look for a cleanser with glycolic or salicylic acid. I also love jojoba oil, which is soothing and great for oily skin because it resembles our own sebum so closely that it signals the body to stop producing oil.

3. **Cleansing balms** with calming ingredients such as glycerin, ceramides, or hyaluronic acid are great for people with sensitive skin. Look for balms with nutrient-rich botanical ingredients like sweet almond oil and cocoa and shea butters,

which melt makeup easily and really soothe the skin. If you opt for a cleansing balm, just know that you don't have to apply it to wet skin; you can put it on dry.

4. **Cream cleansers** are a good fit for people with dry, sensitive skin. These products don't foam, don't leave the skin feeling stripped, and tend to calm the skin after a long day. I recommend using anything that contains soothing ingredients like cocoa or shea butter, or olive, grape seed, or jojoba oil.

Before you wash your face, always wash your hands. If you scrub your face with dirty hands, you're basically spreading germs and bacteria all over your skin. Yuck! Next, rinse your face with lukewarm water and massage your cleanser over your face with your fingertips, using circular motions. This will stimulate your circulation and lymphatic system, getting your cells and lymph moving so your body can repair itself while you sleep. Don't forget to wash your neck as well!

When you're done, blot your face dry with a clean towel. Don't use that dirty towel you've left hanging for two days! It's full of bacteria and mildew. I prefer to use paper towels, simply because I know they're clean.

Your face shouldn't feel squeaky clean after you've washed it. If it does, your cleanser is too acidic, so your skin will overcompensate by producing too much sebum and become oily. Instead, you should feel clean and refreshed and ready to moisturize. Finally, be sure to apply the products you've chosen for steps 2 through 5 within *one minute* of cleansing. Moist skin absorbs products more quickly, so you get more bang for your buck if you act fast.

cleansing products i love

Tatcha Pure One Step Camellia Cleansing Oil: Tatcha makes this amazing cleansing oil that's also a great makeup remover. It easily dissolves waterproof mascara and cleanses your face of makeup and impurities while leaving your skin dewy and glowing. It's also super soothing, so it's perfect for anyone with sensitive skin.

Renée Rouleau Purifying Face Wash: My dear friend and colleague Renée Rouleau makes this amazing foaming face wash that's perfect for oily skin because it cleanses thoroughly without leaving the skin feeling dry or dehydrated.

Honest Beauty Magic Gel-to-Milk Cleanser: My friend Jessica Alba has created so many wonderful things through her company, The Honest Company. I think she's been truly influential worldwide in her quest to create and promote nontoxic, environmentally friendly products for ourselves and our children. Honest Beauty's lovely foaming face wash takes off makeup, doesn't dehydrate, and leaves the skin feeling fresh and clean.

Eve Lom Cleanser: This cleansing balm is the gold standard in the category. Made from four plant-based oils, it does heavy-duty cleansing while improving circulation and bringing glow back to stressed skin.

My own **Vitamin C Face Wash** is a foaming cleanser made for all skin types, and it really cleans without drying the skin. It contains galactoarabinan, a natural substance derived from the larch tree that gently exfoliates and reduces inflammation while also brightening and taking off makeup and surface dirt.

step 2 ● SERUM

Nowadays, serums are everywhere, and they're among my favorite products to use. They're also the second step in your at-home skincare routine because their small molecular composition allows for deep penetration right into your pores.

There's a lot of confusion about serums, however, and the reality is that they are not so easy to understand—not because their formulations are difficult or complex, but because there's very little consistency in terms of their ingredients. There are so many different serums out there that it's hard to say what you should look for and what you should avoid. So, first, let's take a step back and understand the basic form and function of a serum.

Serums are highly concentrated oil or gel formulas. With a multitude of wonderful skin-boosting, -replenishing, and -nourishing ingredients—from vitamin C to argan oil to retinol—serums can moisturize, fight the signs of aging, provide antioxidants, boost collagen, restore skin balance, make the skin more resilient, improve radiance and texture, and much, much more. What makes serums different from most creamy moisturizers is that their ingredients have smaller molecules, so they penetrate more deeply into the layers of the skin. The other great thing about them is that they pack a lot of goodness into one small bottle, so you can typically buy one good serum rather than fifteen different creams to do the same job, allowing you to get the greatest return on your investment.

Any skin type can benefit from a great serum, but if you have dry skin, I recommend looking for one with plant-based oils like argan or jojoba oil, hyaluronic acid for a moisture boost, and

POPPING PIMPLES
JUST. DON'T. DO IT.

If you're cleaning your face and spot a blemish, you might be tempted to pop it. It's just as hard not to scrape off the almost-healed scab that's the result of a pimple you squeezed last week. But when you pick, scrape, or pop anything on your face, you disrupt the skin's protective barrier, which allows harmful germs to invade. Popping a pimple also spreads *P. acnes*, the bacterium inside your pores, across the surrounding area, which in turn may cause more blemishes to form. Further, if you cause yourself to bleed or make any kind of damaging, long-lasting mark on your face, you might develop a scar.

If you have a deep, cystic pimple—an infection under the skin that refuses to come to a head—and you are desperate to do away with it, the first thing to remember is *never* try to extract it yourself. This will only make it worse, as it will irritate the skin and cause it to become more inflamed. Instead, you can apply an ice cube gently to the affected area, which will constrict the blood vessels to reduce redness and swelling. Using a great cleanser that contains salicylic acid and anti-inflammatory ingredients like galactoarabinan will also calm it down and start the healing process.

I remember doing an in-store event some years ago, where I was giving mini facials to the shoppers. A girl walked in with a face full of cystic acne. It was clear she needed immediate relief, so I simply spent ten minutes gently massaging my Vitamin C Face Wash into her skin, being careful not to push on her cysts. After we rinsed her face off, her skin was transformed. While she still had the cysts, they were markedly less noticeable, and her skin was even more toned. Often with cysts, keeping it simple is the best solution! I also *love* treating persistent cystic acne with LED light therapy, which you can get in a salon. But under no circumstances should you pick at your face! A pimple lasts for a few days . . . but scarring can last a lifetime.

omega fatty acids and vitamin C for extra skin nourishment. Oily skin types should look for something water-based, with hyaluronic acid to help hydrate and greens (including algae, broccoli seed oil, kale, and more) to help stimulate the lymphatic system. Finally, sensitive skin types need soothing ingredients, so look for chamomile, calendula, or olive oil, as well as hyaluronic acid or plant-based oils for hydration.

Serums can be used either day or night (or both), and often one can be used in combination with another. Apply a serum on fresh, damp skin within a minute of cleansing. Serums are one of my favorite indulgences, and your skin will thank you for using them. Just research the ingredients carefully and be sure to always wear sunscreen, because serums do not contain it. Otherwise, enjoy!

serums i love

Peach & Lily Glass Skin Refining Serum: My dear friend Alicia Yoon, the founder of Peach & Lily, trusted me with her face for her wedding day. And the truth is, I would trust her with my face any day! Her formulas are impeccable and innovative and offer real results. All of them are good, but her Glass Skin Refining Serum is next level. Full of peptides, soothing fatty acids, hyaluronic acid, and many anti-inflammatories, this serum is a great go-to for all skin types.

Jordan Samuel Skin Hydrate Facial Serum: Jordan Samuel is one of my favorite aestheticians in the beauty universe. A former ballet dancer and all-around rock star, he makes formulas that are simple and easy to love. His Hydrate Facial Serum is light and brightening because it contains hyaluronic acid, vitamin C, peptides (protein parts that help build up collagen, keratin, and elastin), and soothing cucumber.

My own **Daily Serum** is what I call a green juice for the skin. It contains oat grass juice and chlorophyll to de-puff and oxygenate, and hyaluronic acid to super-hydrate. It's light and never too heavy, and it's been my top-selling product worldwide since its launch!

step 3 ● EYE CREAM

Anyone who's ever woken up after a night of restless sleep or dragged themselves out of bed wondering why they had that last stiff drink—or *three*—knows how much of a beating the eye area takes. It has the thinnest skin on the body and doesn't contain any oil glands, so it's no wonder that puffiness, dark circles, and crow's-feet are an issue for many women. In fact, your eyes are one of the first places on your face to show visible signs of aging, starting as soon as your early twenties.

The puffiness around your eyes is due, in part, to inflammation. When you drink too much—either in the long term or over the course of just one night—or eat too many sugary foods, your body becomes inflamed, and that inflammation shows up right away under and around your eyes. Lack of sleep and a diet too high in salt are also major culprits behind puffiness, because our bodies retain water if we're not getting enough rest or are eating too much sodium. While a bad case of raccoon eyes is often due to genetics, dark circles also show up when we don't sleep enough. And they're a telltale sign of aging; as we grow older, we produce less collagen and elastin, so the thin skin in our eye area becomes even more fragile and prone to sagging. As for fine lines? They really can't be avoided. We blink, on average, ten thousand times a day, and that puts our eye area under enormous strain!

Eye cream can work wonders on tired, puffy, wrinkly, or sallow eyes, so when people question whether they *really* need it—or whether they can just use their regular moisturizer—I always insist that eye cream is a *must*. Eye cream is thicker than regular moisturizer because it contains more oil, and that gives a major boost to dry, dehydrated eyes. Eye creams also contain more targeted ingredients than regular moisturizers. I love products with cucumber because it de-puffs and tightens; lactic acid, which promotes cell turnover; and peptides, which support elasticity. Retinol can also help cell turnover, and caffeine constricts blood vessels, which decreases puffiness. A lot of people love to refrigerate their eye cream because cold also helps restrict blood flow (and it feels great on your skin). Just don't put your eye cream—or any product—in the freezer, because extreme cold can damage the layers of the skin.

You should use eye cream in the morning and at night, after serum and before moisturizer. Using your fourth finger—the weakest digit, so you won't press too hard—pat cream lightly onto your eye area, working from the inside out. Resist the urge to rub it in; this part of your face is just too delicate for that. Don't forget the corners of your eyes, either. I promise you that within two weeks of regular use, eye cream will make you appear years younger. Couple that with enough sleep, a good diet, and not too much alcohol, and you'll look like you've traveled back in time!

eye creams i love

Goldfaden MD Bright Eyes: This wonderful eye cream contains vitamin K to help with darkness, peptides for firming, and jojoba oil to soothe the delicate eye area.

Renée Rouleau Total Eye Repair Cream firms and repairs the skin while at the same time giving a hydrating boost to the delicate eye area.

My Revitalizing Eye Cream de-puffs and strengthens the connective tissue with cucumber and oat amino protein while also hydrating the skin. The cream's rich combination of zinc, magnesium, and potassium stimulates the lymphatic system.

INGREDIENT SPOTLIGHT: ACIDS

Put acid on my skin? You gotta be kidding me! The startled reaction many of my clients have when I mention the word "acid" is no surprise, because it conjures up images of burning, searing, blistered flesh. Ouch! But that is *not* what acids are all about. It's quite the opposite: acids are vital ingredients in many of the beauty products I recommend, including creams, serums, toners, and more.

In scientific terms, an acid is a chemical substance made up of molecules that neutralize alkaline substances. Acids change the chemical composition of your skin cells, breaking down or dissolving the bonds between living cells and those that are dead so the dead cells can be shed. This "out with the old" approach allows new, fresh, strong skin cells to develop, and that leads to brighter, younger, healthier-looking skin.

There are hundreds of different kinds of acids out there. Some come in the form of peels, some are vitamins, some are serums, and some give us extra hydration—but whatever their form, acids are skincare essentials. Most of the acids you'll find are mixed with other ingredients to balance them, creating a gentle yet effective way to improve your skin, often dramatically. Here are some of the common acids you'll find in skincare products:

INGREDIENT SPOTLIGHT: ACIDS

Alpha hydroxy acids: There are many different kinds of alpha hydroxy acids (AHAs), but the most popular ones are lactic and glycolic acid. **Lactic acid** is derived from souring milk, and it's one of the milder AHAs, with a larger molecular structure that has difficulty penetrating the skin layers below the epidermis. Since the time of the ancient Egyptians, lactic acid has been used to dissolve dead skin cells, lightly exfoliate, and balance the skin's pH level. It also clears out toxins and debris, boosts the production of collagen—the protein that gives structure to your skin—and deeply hydrates the skin. Over time, it can also help reduce fine lines and wrinkles. Lactic acid is a very popular ingredient in many gentle peels and mild exfoliants, and in very little time, it'll help leave your skin baby soft. (As a side note, if you have a dairy allergy or sensitivity, do not worry about using lactic acid on your skin. Those with lactose intolerance typically only have issues if they ingest dairy or dairy-derived substances.)

Glycolic acid is derived from sugarcane, and it has a smaller molecular structure than lactic acid, so it can travel through the epidermis and into the dermis. This deep penetration makes it a bit harsher than lactic acid, so if you have extremely sensitive skin, please use it sparingly or test it out before incorporating it into your daily routine. Glycolic acid is one of the most popular ingredients in chemical peels, because it's so powerful in promoting cell turnover. It also stimulates collagen production, which helps eliminate fine lines and wrinkles and gives you an overall more youthful, brighter, more plumped-up appearance.

Salicylic acid: The one and only beta hydroxy acid, salicylic acid is most commonly found in acne-fighting products. While it can penetrate the layers of the skin as well as glycolic acid and lactic acid, it's also oil-soluble, which means that when it gets into your pores, it dissolves the gunky dead skin cells inside them, effectively unclogging them. Even if you don't have acne or aren't prone to breakouts, it's a terrific acid for mild peels because it helps even out the oily patches many of us have on our skin. It's also anti-inflammatory, which makes it safe for daily use, even for people with very sensitive skin.

Hyaluronic acid: This substance is produced naturally by our skin cells to help regulate moisture levels. It helps your cells hold in water, causing you to look plump, refreshed, and pillow soft. Unfortunately, the amount of hyaluronic acid your body produces decreases as you age, and over time—coupled with environmental stressors like pollution and sun exposure—this causes your skin to sag, flake, or look dull or uneven. That's where beauty products can be so effective. Unlike other acids, hyaluronic acid doesn't dissolve dead skin cells, so you can't use it as an exfoliant. But no matter your skin type, you can enjoy its antioxidant properties, which shield the body against environmental free radicals that can damage the skin, and you can use it daily.

Amino acids: These compounds within your cells help build protein and synthesize hormones and neurotransmitters. Your skin is primarily made

INGREDIENT SPOTLIGHT: ACIDS

up of proteins, so you can probably guess that amino acids are a *must*. The problem is that of the twenty amino acids your body needs to function, it makes only eleven, so you have to get the other nine through diet or supplements. Using beauty products that contain amino acids isn't a replacement for consuming protein-rich foods, but these products can complement a healthy diet, helping your skin cells bind water molecules and move moisture throughout the skin. Amino acids also perform the dual function of acting as antioxidants and helping the body *create* more antioxidants. I recommend looking for the following amino acids in products: proline, leucine, glycine, arginine, lysine, histidine, methionine, and serine. Amino acids are also the building blocks of **peptides**, which are fragments of protein that signal your cells to produce more collagen, elastin, and keratin. With more of these essential substances in your skin, it becomes firmer, plumper, more elastic, and more youthful-looking. As far as I'm concerned, you can't have too many peptides in your skin cells, so no matter what your skin type is, look for products containing them.

Omega fatty acids: These are naturally occurring acids found in many of the foods we eat, including fish and a host of plant, bean, and fruit oils. However, they're not often discussed in terms of the amazing benefits they offer as skincare ingredients. Trust me, they can work wonders! Fatty acids help reinforce skin cells' membranes, essentially creating stronger cells. This, in turn, protects the skin against moisture loss and environmental stress. Fatty acids also soothe and hydrate the skin, making them perfect for people with dry, sensitive skin. When you're scanning the beauty aisles, look for oleic, palmitic, linoleic, and linolenic acids.

Kojic acid: A gentle chemical derived from mushrooms, this is another acid I love. It's used in exfoliants, serums, cleansers, and moisturizers, and helps decrease melanin production and even the skin tone.

Alpha-lipoic acid: Also known as ALA, this is found in spinach, broccoli, and potatoes. Rich in antioxidants, it's wonderfully anti-inflammatory.

Mandelic acid: This is a milder alpha hydroxy peel that's great for sensitive skin because it's made up of bigger molecules than glycolic acid, so it penetrates into the skin more slowly.

Ascorbic acid and retinoic acid: Two of the most popular and well-known acids found in skincare products and treatments. For more information on ascorbic acid (also known as vitamin C), see page 24; for more on retinoic acid (similar to retinol), turn to page 120. But for now, know that in the right products and with the right skin type, they can each be terrific!

INGREDIENT SPOTLIGHT: ACIDS

products with acids i love

Sunday Riley Good Genes All-In-One Lactic Acid Treatment: This fabulous product has the ability to even out the pigment in your skin, brighten, and soothe, all while giving you a righteous peel.

Allies of Skin Mandelic Pigmentation Corrector Night Serum: Mandelic acid is an alpha hydroxy acid, but it's gentler than many other AHAs like glycolic acid. This is a powerful serum that reduces blackheads, keeps blemishes away, and increases cell turnover while boosting and strengthening the skin with essential peptides.

The Organic Pharmacy Four Acid Peel: This is an awesome little fruit peel formula that uses glycolic, lactic, citric, and tartaric acids to gently exfoliate the skin. I'm obsessed because it's a major results-oriented formula, but its ingredients are safe and pure.

Tatcha The Rice Polish: Classic: This foaming enzyme powder made from Japanese rice bran is an absolute skincare star. You pour a little bit in your hand and add water to activate it. It completely resurfaces even the most delicate skin without damaging.

My own **Dawn Face Mask** is a combination of vitamin C and mandelic acid and is perfect for anyone who struggles with breakouts and needs to even out the surface of the skin.

step 4 ● MOISTURIZE

Most of the women I see in my salons believe they understand how to moisturize. They think: *What could be so hard? All you do is slather on a cream or oil (or both!) right after you wash your face, morning and night.* They've been doing the same thing the same way for years, and in some ways, their process is just fine. However, most of my clients don't understand *why* it's so essential to moisturize and exactly *what* they should look for in a moisturizer. With thousands and thousands of creams, oils, and serums on the market, it's also hard to cut through the jargon and choose the right ingredients. I'm here to help.

I'm going to say something controversial first: not everyone needs to use moisturizer. I've met men and women with very oily complexions for whom moisturizing will cause more breakouts than they already get. Instead of recommending products, I tell these people to look for the dietary and lifestyle culprits for their excessively oily skin. If they address those issues, after a few weeks, they can tiptoe into moisturizing by testing out a very light serum or facial oil. If eliminating certain foods or behaviors doesn't stop their breakouts, though, they should focus on trying out new ways to cleanse, exfoliate, tone, and soothe their skin.

you should always use a separate sun protectant in addition to—and after—moisturizer. The other reason is that a moisturizer with sunscreen probably doesn't offer strong enough protection to defend against the sun. In a July 2018 study, researchers from the University of Liverpool found that when moisturizer alone is used for sun protection, people miss an average of 16 percent of their face, especially around the eyes. If sunscreen is used alone, they only neglect 11 percent of their face. Further, people tend to apply a thinner layer of moisturizer, while they slather on sunscreen a little thicker.

Always look for a moisturizer in opaque packaging (rather than clear glass or plastic) because many of the wonderful ingredients I mentioned above can break down when exposed to sunlight.

moisturizers i love

Peach & Lily Matcha Pudding Antioxidant Cream ● For dry skin, this lightweight, gentle cream is amazing and provides super hydration all day long. I like it because it's loaded with antioxidants to help protect the skin from the stressors we face daily, while hydrating at the same time.

Renée Rouleau Daily Mattifying Solution ● Perfect for oily skin, this very lightweight lotion helps reduce shine and lessens inflammation from breakouts. It also has antibacterial properties to assist with healing.

Burt's Bees Daily Moisturizing Cream (Sensitive) ● This inexpensive cream is perfect for anyone who has a bit of sensitivity or full-blown eczema. It has cotton extract to help protect the skin against environmental stressors, and it also soothes and gives a moisture boost.

My Daily Hydrating Cream contains avocado oil to provide vital B vitamins to your skin while hydrating it. Shea and cocoa butters melt at body temperature and are absorbed into the skin, so it feels perfectly balanced and not sticky.

● ● ●

INGREDIENT SPOTLIGHT: ANTIOXIDANTS

"Antioxidant" is one of those words that you see in beauty articles and on food labels all the time, yet if I stopped you on the street and asked you to define it, you'd be stumped. Allow me to pull back the curtain on these often-misunderstood substances and show you why they're so essential to your skin's health, how to use them, and why, when it comes to antioxidants, there *can* be too much of a good thing.

Simply put, antioxidants are molecules that donate electrons to free radicals, stabilizing them and combatting their damaging effects. Some antioxidants are produced by our bodies, while others, like vitamin C, vitamin E, and flavonoids, are found in foods. While antioxidants exist in almost all plant- and animal-based ingredients, the foods that contain the highest concentration include grapes, berries, nuts (especially walnuts and Brazil nuts), dark green vegetables, sweet potatoes, green tea, beans, and whole grains. While vitamin supplements containing antioxidants are popular, there's no evidence that super-high doses are beneficial to your health.

Antioxidants have long been known to reverse the signs of aging—especially wrinkles and dark spots—when applied directly to your skin. But which types of antioxidants should you look for in the products you buy? I recommend **vitamin C**, which evens pigmentation, increases elasticity, brightens your complexion, and improves your skin's resilience. I also like **vitamin E**, which boosts collagen. I recommend looking for a particular type of vitamin E called alpha-tocopherol, which penetrates the skin more easily than other forms of the vitamin. Additional antioxidant-rich substances include green tea, lycopene, red palm oil, cocoa butter, African honey, coffee berry, lutein, beta-carotene, selenium, alpha-lipoic acid, and gluthathione. These ingredients can be found in many of my favorite products.

But just as with supplements, you can overdo it with serums and creams that are supercharged with antioxidants. Too much of one particular substance can lead to cell damage, so you need a diverse range of antioxidants in combination with substances such as ceramides, hyaluronic acid, glycerin, retinol, peptides, and niacinamide.

Finally, antioxidants break down in light and when they're exposed to air. If you're looking for an antioxidant-rich serum or cream, make sure it comes in an opaque package that, when opened, won't let in too much oxygen. Don't buy a product in a jar; instead, look for a bottle with a medicine dropper or a dispenser with a narrow pump.

antioxidant products i love

Paula's Choice 10% Niacinamide Booster: Paula's Choice is probably one of the best resources for skincare out there. Their niacinamide serum gives the epidermis a great protective boost of vitamin B_3, which reduces fine lines, prevents hyperpigmentation, and is a natural anti-inflammatory.

Drunk Elephant C-Firma Day Serum: This is a great combination of vitamin C for protection and healing and a nice hyaluronic acid boost for hydration.

stepping out the door on a cloudy day, or just walking down your driveway to get the newspaper, you should use it. Why? Because 80 percent of the sun's rays make it through clouds, even in the winter, and 85 percent reflect off ice, pavement, sand, and water, meaning wearing a hat without sun protection at the beach isn't enough. Again, sun damage is cumulative—that is, if you get ten minutes here and twenty minutes the next day, you've still sustained thirty solid minutes of sun damage. That's thirty minutes too many.

Some of the questions I get asked by clients most frequently are about sunscreen—they want to know how to choose one that is safe, and which products I recommend. Before I can address those questions, let's look at the two categories of sunscreens: chemical and mineral.

Chemical sunscreens are those that contain synthetic ingredients, including oxybenzone, Mexoryl, avobenzone, octisalate, octocrylene, homosalate, and octinoxate. People use the term "chemical," but this is misleading, because many of the ingredients are carbon-based, or organic. Instead of blocking the sun's UVA and UVB rays (UVA rays penetrate into the dermis, while UVB rays burn the skin's surface), these ingredients absorb light like a sponge, causing a chemical reaction within the skin, which then releases the rays as heat. These sunscreens are simpler to use because they are thinner in texture and easier to spread on the skin's surface. Chemical sunscreens penetrate the skin cells, so they need time to soak in, which is why you need to apply them thirty minutes before sun exposure.

Mineral-based sunscreens contain titanium dioxide or zinc oxide, ingredients that sit on the top of the skin and deflect the sun's rays. As a bonus, these two ingredients have been shown to promote healing in the skin and in wounds. They also begin to protect against the sun immediately upon application and are noncomedogenic, meaning their molecules are so large they won't clog your pores. While mineral-based sunscreens go on a little thicker than chemical sunscreens, many brands now mix in silicone to deliver a smoother finish, so you won't look like a ghost if you use them.

You should always use sunscreen in addition to moisturizer, putting it on just after your skin has absorbed the moisturizer so the sunscreen sits on top of the epidermis for maximum effect. Finally, if you use a spray sunscreen, be sure to apply it liberally and rub it in thoroughly; unlike creams, sprays often don't provide even coverage.

The bottom line is, always wear sunscreen, but do your research and be very selective about the products you use. Sun damage is the number one reason for prematurely aging skin, not to mention elevated cancer risk. So please, protect yourself wisely. It's worth the investment.

sunscreens i love

Nuxe Sun Melting Spray for Face and Body: This is a new obsession of mine. I love all of Nuxe's body products, but their sunscreen is amazing. Their high-protection SPF 50 is an easy-on, easy-to-reapply spray that protects against UVA and UVB rays.

MDSolarSciences Mineral Moisture Defense: MDSolarSciences is probably my favorite sunscreen line, offering both chemical and physical blocks. I love the Mineral Moisture Defense SPF 50, which goes on easily even though it's a mineral-based sunscreen. It's also excellent protection for people like me who tend to develop melasma on the face.

add-ons for your routine

In addition to your five-step daily routine, there are some terrific (and, dare I say, life-changing) techniques and products that you can use a few times a week or as little as once or twice a month to enhance the quality of your skin. As you read through the list that follows, you may find some products—for example, a retinol cream or an exfoliant—that you are currently using daily. If these products or treatments are harsh on your skin, consider treating them as extras that you cycle into your routine only as needed.

Let's take a closer look at what these extras entail.

DRY BRUSHING

You brush your teeth twice a day without batting an eyelash—it's part of your routine, you've always done it, and you wouldn't skip it if you dared. It's time to think of dry brushing in the same way. Dry brushing has been around for centuries, but in the past few years, it's gained tremendous popularity. Given that it takes less than a minute and requires a tool that usually costs less than $10, I hope everyone embraces it!

YOUR TOWEL
IS A BEAUTY
PRODUCT, TOO!

Towels may be the most overlooked and misunderstood component of a good skincare routine. Almost every client I meet is using the wrong kind of towel, the wrong way, both to cleanse and dry their skin.

Let's start with cleansing. Most people who use washcloths to wash their skin use the terry cloth variety. Terry cloth can be incredibly abrasive, so as you move it across your face, you're exfoliating at the same time you're cleansing. The fabric's tiny "fingers" also pull at the skin, leading to sagginess over time. Finally, the harshness of the fabric can strip your skin of essential oils, making it dry even if you properly moisturize. The good news is that there are dozens of different types of cleansing cloths on the market—I especially love bamboo, muslin, or soft cotton towels. Eve Lom Muslin Cloths are one of my favorite towels for washing my face. They gently exfoliate while you cleanse and really help remove all your makeup. As with any towel, use them to wash your face gently and slowly, moving them in circular, upward strokes on both sides of your face and neck.

Facial cloths are a breeding ground for bacteria, fungus, mold, and mildew, and they can quickly become full of any of those nasty things, plus dead skin cells and environmental debris. I recommend using them only once, then washing them or throwing them out if they're disposable. If you have acne, try paper towels instead of regular towels to dry your face so you don't spread bacteria, and throw out the paper towel when you're finished with it. If you're not prone to breakouts, you can probably get away with using a face towel twice or even three times, but don't hang it up to dry, use it several more times, and then toss it in the wash only when it begins to smell. Yuck!

When it comes time to dry your skin, don't reach for the towel you use on the rest of your body after a shower. It's not just that towels are full of germs, mold, mildew, and yeast; they also contain traces of the other products you apply to your body, like shampoos, fragrances, and soap. The ingredients in these products can irritate your skin or clog your pores. Use a separate towel of any kind—including terry cloth—but simply pat your skin dry rather than rubbing it. I like to use paper towels to blot; that way I don't have to remember to wash my towels every day (or every few days, if you're not prone to breakouts).

Finally, if you do plan to use a towel more than once—either for cleansing or drying—hang it outside the bathroom to dry. Even a well-ventilated bathroom can be far more humid than other rooms, meaning it takes longer for towels to dry, leading to the growth of mold, mildew, or yeast.

Not only does dry brushing gently exfoliate dead skin and increase circulation, it also increases collagen production. It drains excess water out of your tissues, making you look less puffy and bloated. And it gives your skin a little workout, making it thicker and more resilient, which helps to reduce the appearance of cellulite toward the surface of your skin.

Dry brushing is as straightforward and simple as it sounds; all you need is a natural-fiber, firm-bristled brush, which should be available in almost all drugstores and online. Some people prefer a brush without a handle, but given that you should brush all parts of your body, including your back, I prefer one with a long handle.

Before you begin brushing, your body should be completely dry and free of any products. I like to dry brush before a shower simply because I can immediately wash off any dead skin when I'm done brushing, but you may prefer to do it right before bed as a way to relax. Whatever you decide, take the brush firmly in your hand and brush in short, upward strokes toward your heart, applying firm yet gentle pressure so you don't irritate your skin. In order to make sure you don't miss any part of your body, start at your feet and work your way up your legs. As you move on to your arms—making sure to brush your underarms—you'll notice how warm you feel. That's because, like a massage, dry

glow from within

brushing increases your circulation. Brush your backside, your back, your tummy, your neck, and your chest. You can skip your face; it's a sensitive area, and you can exfoliate it with a gentle product instead.

Voilà! Dry brushing your whole body should take less than a minute, and it will become like second nature within a few days. The more you do anything in beauty, the bigger the payoff, so I do it every day for maximum results, but even brushing just twice a week will have visible benefits. Just be sure you wash your brush with baby shampoo or a gentle soap every two weeks; you don't want dead skin accumulating in the brush, which will not only make your brush dirty and smelly, but could lead to bacterial growth, too. As you do with your towel, hang it outside your bathroom to dry.

If you dry brush every day, I promise you'll see noticeable results within two weeks. When I started dry brushing my body, I was preparing for my wedding and was trying every beauty treatment and routine I could think of. I knew dry brushing would be an amazing way to maintain elasticity and reduce cellulite, but the results were beyond what I could have imagined. In two weeks, my booty looked two inches higher than it had when I started! Pretty amazing for something so simple, right?

dry brushes i love

My dry brush is called the **Ritual Brush,** but any traditional natural-bristle brush will work!

EPIDERMAL GROWTH FACTORS/STEM CELLS

Around 2015, epidermal growth factors (EGFs) was one of the buzziest terms in skincare, and this mysterious-sounding ingredient began popping up in everything from masks to serums to moisturizers. The truth is that EGFs—large proteins that occur naturally in our cells and in plant cells—are nothing new. They've been known as stem cells for two decades, and they were discovered by a biologist and a biochemist in 1986. Their findings—which showed that EGFs could stimulate skin growth at the cellular level, therefore speeding the healing of wounds—was so extraordinary and groundbreaking that the two scientists won a Nobel Prize!

EGFs are found in all kinds of bodily fluids—like urine, breast milk, blood, and saliva—and are abundant in wounds, where they're working hard to regenerate tissue and help you heal. EGFs exist in all the various types of skin cells found in the dermis and epidermis—from keratinocytes (which form keratin) to melanocytes (which form pigment). EGFs direct these cells to grow, divide, repair, and turn over, and that leads to the production of more collagen, keratin, and elastin.

Unfortunately, when you turn thirty, your EGF levels begin to decline. That means your skin cells don't turn over as fast as they used to, causing your skin to sag; become thin; form fine lines, wrinkles, and circles under the eyes; and look dry, dull, or lifeless. You may be shocked to hear that when you're eighteen, your skin cells renew every two to three weeks. At forty, it's every forty-five to sixty days! But thanks to the EGFs that have been added to many beauty products, you can fight all these unpleasant side effects of aging.

The EGFs you find in beauty products are derived from human stem cells, made from genetically engineered barley seeds, or derived from any number of plants including irises, coneflowers, green Swiss apples, raspberries, grapes, and roses. Before you become concerned that the use of stem cells crosses a moral line for you—or that anyone suffered or died so you could have your wrinkles erased—rest assured that that's *not* the case. The stem cells that helped produce EGFs in many product lines were derived from a single cell culture from a donated piece of human tissue. Let me repeat: it was a willingly given single cell from a piece of unwanted tissue that would have otherwise gone to waste. If you use these products, you are simply applying the protein derived from that tissue—not the tissue itself.

The best and most popular type of stem cells comes from a very rare Swiss apple that was cultivated over three hundred years ago for its long storage life. Today, scientists extract the stem cells of this fruit to use in skincare, and they do a remarkable job of helping to reverse the signs of aging, increasing the life of skin cells, and stimulating new skin cell generation. In clinical testing, this ingredient causes wrinkle reduction by 15 percent in just four weeks' time.

While other studies backing the efficacy of EGFs are still limited (and most used sample groups of fewer than one hundred people), they're not to be ignored. In a trial for one company, twenty-nine women who applied an EGF serum to one side of their face twice a day for eight weeks saw the thickness of their facial skin increase by 60 percent on that side. Based on my own experience, I've seen a noticeable difference in my clients' complexions after applying EGFs. They're more luminous, radiant, plump, and elastic, and they have fewer fine lines and wrinkles. Some studies have reported that people may experience psoriasis or irritation because EGFs force their skin cells into overdrive, but in my experience, this only happens in a small percentage of people.

I once had a client who got a bad sunburn at her bachelorette party, just one week before her bridal shower. When she came in for a facial, she was desperate for help. Most facialists focus only on the face, but I like to address the skin as a whole. While I gave my client a Super Nova Facial to rehydrate her skin and plump it back up so it would look bright, healthy, and young again, I thought about what to do with the damaged skin on the rest of her body. I reached for a few of my Twilight Masks—which contain EGFs—and started covering her whole body with them. We kept them on for a whole hour, and when we took them off, her skin looked nothing more than slightly sun-kissed. She was hydrated, glowing, and ready to be photographed!

Products containing EGFs should be applied to dry skin once a week right after cleansing, and you should be careful not to pair them with an acidic substance like vitamin C or alpha hydroxy acids, which can break down the amino acid chain. Otherwise, enjoy the amazing benefits that modern science has produced as you discover how EGFs can help you turn back years on the clock!

egf products i love

Nurse Jamie EGF Botanical Complex: Jamie is a friend of many of my friends, although I've never had the pleasure of meeting her. I love this light hydrating serum that contains plant stem cells, EGFs, and phospholipids, which reduce the signs of aging.

DNA Intensive Renewal: This EGF formula is loaded with peptides, vitamin E, and enzymes, and has everything you need to make your skin glow! It's also good for all skin types, which I particularly love.

My Twilight Face Mask is the most healing product I have in my line. I remember once putting it on my skin after I had been injured pretty badly from a fall. Before I applied the mask, my skin was red and raw, but after, it looked like nothing had happened. It was remarkable!

EXFOLIATING

Few things feel better than skin that's as soft and smooth as velvet. That's why I *love* exfoliating! But as with any skincare ritual, you have to strike the right balance with the right products. Your skin is delicate, so be careful never to overdo it when it comes to exfoliating.

Exfoliation is an essential part of a beauty routine for several reasons. First, your skin is your body's first line of defense—in fact, it's arguably the most important component of your immune system—and it endures a tremendous amount of abuse. At all hours, whether you're inside or outside, pollution, dirt, bacteria, food particles, viruses, and any number of foreign agents come into contact with your skin cells. When they do, your cells expend a lot of energy fighting infection, and many die. Exfoliation ensures that new skin cells can come to the surface and that dirt and old skin won't clog your pores. Second, over time—and especially because of sun exposure—our skin doesn't slough off old, dead cells as easily. That's why babies and children have such gorgeous, supple skin; their skin cells are constantly shedding and regenerating, giving them a youthful glow.

There are two routes you can take with exfoliation: using an abrasive material to physically remove old cells, or using an acid-based system. I like both—choose either method, based on your own preferences.

If you do choose to exfoliate with a scrub, make sure it's a fine-grained scrub. The exfoliating mask I produce is made of pumice, which has an almost soft, sandlike feel to it. Other scrubs I recommend use sugar, which doesn't irritate the skin. Many conventional, inexpensive exfoliants used to contain plastic microbeads, but they are terrible for the environment—killing fish populations and clogging the water supply with harmful plastic.

Thankfully, there is now a full ban against them in the US, Canada, France, New Zealand, and a handful of other regions.

I can't stress enough that you should use something *gentle* to exfoliate. Some substances like apricot kernels or walnut shells have uneven surfaces, and these can tear the stratum corneum, the outermost layer of the epidermis. The stratum corneum keeps moisture in and foreign agents out, so if you rip it, you won't just be at risk of getting an infection, your skin may also look dull or flaky. Furthermore, exfoliating harshly if you have a pimple or are prone to breakouts may pop the pimple under the surface of the skin, spreading bacteria and causing an even bigger breakout.

Acid scrubs are also quite popular with good reason; they help you remove dead skin cells without any risk of skin tearing. Look for an acid-based exfoliating scrub with glycolic, lactic, or salicylic acid as its primary active ingredient. All three are great at smoothing your skin, evening tone, eliminating small bumps, increasing hydration, and diminishing the look of wrinkles, but glycolic and lactic acids are recommended for dry skin, while salicylic acid is best for oily skin. Secondary ingredients can include citric, malic, or tartaric acids. (To learn more about acids and their benefits to skincare, see page 79.)

Exfoliate *after cleansing*, using either your clean fingers or a cotton pad, working in an upward direction and moving in small

glow from within

circles. You don't have to wait for an acid scrub to dry before you put on cream. Just be sure not to skip applying sunscreen if you're heading outside, as your exfoliated skin may be extra sensitive. No matter what kind of scrub you choose, you should exfoliate at least twice a week, especially in summer when humidity causes more pollutants to stick to your skin. Be careful not to exfoliate more than three times a week, however, because this could cause irritation or sensitivity. You should also only exfoliate at home, rather than in a public place like the gym, where there's more bacteria on surfaces, and where you could contract an infection.

Regardless, enjoy how great you'll feel after exfoliating. A great scrub stimulates collagen, promotes cell turnover, reduces puffiness, and makes your skin positively glow.

exfoliating products i love

ARCONA Cranberry Gommage: I love the feel of buffing away all my dead skin cells and impurities. This scrub is loaded with antioxidants, so it brightens and boosts the skin's strength. It also smells delicious and is full of wonderful ingredients.

Goldfaden MD Doctor's Scrub: This scrub uses ruby crystals to gently slough off dead skin cells while infusing the skin with balancing jojoba oil, seaweed extract for boosting detoxification, and hyaluronic acid for light hydration.

My **Exfoliating Mask** contains pumice for a gentle scrub (perfect for your T-zone) and pineapple enzymes and lactic acid to provide all-over brightening and resurfacing. Leave it on for at least five minutes and up to overnight to make you glow all over. We call it a "facial in a jar"!

MASKS

I *love* masks. They're the perfect combination of pampering and skin rejuvenation, providing a host of ways to improve your skin's tone, texture, hydration, and more. People often assume that masks only offer short-term benefits—such as hydrating, unclogging pores, or exfoliating—but my decades of experience (both personal and professional!) have shown me that if you use a mask at least twice a week, your skin will dramatically improve over time.

There are a dizzying number and variety of masks on the market, though, so I'll do my best to show you what you should look for.

•   •   •

glow from within

Clay masks are terrific for people with oily or acne-prone skin because they pull out impurities, unclogging your pores and giving your skin a cleaner, fresher look. They also rebalance your oil production, so if you have combination skin, they'll help the oily areas become less so. In addition, clay is beneficial for the lymphatic system because it helps your skin cells flush out toxins. If your skin is looking especially dull or tired, a clay mask will help brighten it. One of my favorite types of clay is kaolin clay, made from the mineral kaolinite, which leaves your skin feeling smooth, exfoliated, hydrated, and mattified.

Sheet masks are so popular that you can't leave a beauty store without seeing fifteen different varieties at the checkout aisle, selling for anywhere from fifty cents to fifty dollars per mask. I love sheet masks because there is a tailored product for every individual's skincare goal, whether that's hydrating, soothing, fighting blemishes, or brightening. I always recommend that my clients use masks after exfoliating to get maximum penetration into the skin. Some of my staff members even sleep in them! Sheet masks are also great for people on the go. I travel frequently, and every time I get on a plane, I put on a sheet mask, close my eyes, and relax while my skin is protected from the dehydrating air inside the cabin. If I startle one of the flight attendants or my fellow passengers, I just smile and hand them one of my masks to enjoy at home! Finally, sheet masks are so easy to use. After cleansing and/or exfoliating, you just open the package, peel off the backing, and place one on your face, pressing from the center to the edges. Leave the mask on for twenty minutes; when you take it off, there's really no need to rinse or cleanse again. Just rub the soothing, hydrating ingredients into your face and neck, and follow with your regular serum, moisturizer, and eye cream routine.

Cream masks are great for dry or sensitive skin, or for people who are concerned with the effects of aging. With ingredients like avocado oil, shea butter, or any number of fatty acids, a cream mask will help your skin feel plumper and dewier. If you're prone to breakouts or acne, though, this may not be the best mask choice for you. The intensely hydrating oils they contain may clog pores and lead to breakouts.

No matter what kind of mask you choose, it's okay to leave it on overnight if your skin can tolerate it. (Though sheet masks may slip off!) Nighttime is your skin's opportunity to repair itself, and if you let the ingredients soak in while you sleep, your skin will look terrific in the morning. When you wake up, keep your regular routine of cleansing (if you wash in the morning), then applying serum, eye cream, and moisturizer. It's also okay to switch up the type of mask you use—both in terms of the type of mask and ingredients. But because there are thousands upon thousands of ingredients to choose from, I'll try to simplify them based on your skin's needs.

If you're prone to **acne**, you need ingredients that will help your skin redistribute oils. Charcoal, zinc, and probiotics (such as those found in yogurt) are good ingredients to seek out.

If your skin is just a bit **clogged with blackheads**, consider those same ingredients, but you might also look for an exfoliating mask, especially if it contains volcanic rock.

For those of you with **dry skin**, search for masks that include hyaluronic acid, avocado oil, yogurt, shea butter, collagen, algae, or peptides.

If you have **fine lines**, consider masks with epidermal growth factors, antioxidants, and some hydrating ingredient such as those listed above for dry skin.

●　●　●

If your skin is **dull**, try glycolic acid or galactoarabinan, both of which help with cell turnover. As your skin regenerates, you'll see improvements with your pesky wrinkles and fine lines.

If you have **sensitive skin,** look for chamomile, aloe, arnica, or sulfur, all of which have soothing, anti-inflammatory qualities. I recommend using sheet masks rather than other types, too, because they have fewer preservatives that might irritate your skin.

Finally, if you have **oily skin**, try clay masks with zinc and jojoba oil, which help tell the skin to stop producing so much oil.

Now sit back, relax, and put on a mask!

masks i love

Dr. Hauschka Clarifying Clay Mask: Dr. Hauschka has been doing clean beauty for decades, and in my mind, they're still the gold standard for pure skincare that really works. I love his Clarifying Clay Mask, which draws out impurities and soothes with witch hazel. It's great for oily skin or breakouts.

• • •

glow from within

Caudalie Moisturizing Mask: This mask has lovely grape seed oil and Vinolevure (an extract from wine yeast) to help infuse the skin with essential antioxidants, which makes it positively glow!

Peach & Lily Good Skin Drench + Nourish Sheet Mask: Each of these sheet masks contain a laundry list of great ingredients, and your skin will instantly look better and brighter after one use.

Peach & Lily Lavender Bedside Mask: This nighttime mask is awesome because it's scented with lavender to help you fall asleep. It also provides gentle exfoliation with lactic acid, salicylic acid, and milk proteins. It hydrates, calms, and brightens skin overnight.

My Forever Glow Anti-Aging Face Sheet Mask is one of my bestsellers. It contains hyaluronic acid for hydration and peptides for elasticity, and gives you an instant overall glow.

OILS

Many of my clients are hesitant to try oils because they assume they'll be too greasy, heavy, or pore-clogging for their skin, but nothing could be further from the truth. Facial oils—which may be an ingredient in a serum you use daily, or a standalone product to be used under moisturizer—help control sebum production, reduce inflammation, and are refreshing, hydrating, and skin replenishing. Their many benefits make them a perfect complement to your skincare routine—no matter what type of skin you have. Personally, I can't live without an oil on my skin at all times!

I remember one client who came to see me many years ago with red, raw skin. She was what I would call a "laser abuser"—her dermatologist had urged her to do a laser or chemical peel every six weeks, but she was only twenty-eight and those treatments were *way* too harsh for her young skin! Her goal was to preserve her youthful glow, but in reality, those "preventive measures" were thinning and aging her skin, making it so inflamed that it reacted to everything it came in contact with. My solution was very simple: in addition to doing LED light treatments on a weekly basis, I suggested she use one of my oil serums night and day. At first, she was hesitant, but I asked her to give it a month. Sure enough, one month later, she looked like a different person. Her skin was less red and less reactive, and she looked years younger than she had the day I met her.

There are two types of facial oils: plant-based oils, which are

glow from within

usually derived from pressing, and essential oils, which are obtained through a distillation process.

You may be familiar with **essential oils** from aromatherapy, massage, or that moment in yoga class when your teacher gently rubs your temples with a soothing oil, making you ten times more relaxed than you were before. *Namaste.* Essential oils like lavender, rose, bergamot, orange, lemon, bitter orange, and peppermint smell absolutely divine and offer some medicinal benefits, but I'm not crazy about using most of them on your face. These oils can be quite potent, and their chemical composition changes when exposed to sunlight or oxygen, which can cause skin irritation. Some essential oils may also disrupt your skin's microbiome, triggering an allergic response like eczema. So skip the smelly stuff. You don't really need it anywhere near your face.

Plant-derived facial oils are light easily absorbed, and will give your face an instant shiny, hydrated glow. My number one face oil recommendation is **jojoba oil**, which is rich in zinc, copper, and vitamins B and E. It has a chemical composition similar to that of your skin's natural sebum, so almost anyone can use it and enjoy the dewiness it instantly delivers. Another favorite of mine is **argan oil**, which is derived from the seeds of the Moroccan argan tree. (Fun fact: The seed kernels used to make pure argan oil have passed through the bodies of goats who climbed up the argan trees and ate their fruit! Local women then extract the oil in an age-old practice that's considered an art form.) Argan oil is high in vitamin E, omega-3 fatty acids, and antioxidants, and helps build up cell membranes, increase collagen, and calm the skin. Unfortunately, it can feel too drying for some people, so I recommend looking for a serum that combines argan oil with other oils to balance it out. For example, my Rejuvenating Serum has argan, olive, rose hip seed (for improving circulation), jojoba, and neroli oils (for protection again cell mutations caused by the sun).

Avocado oil is excellent for chronically dry, irritated, or sensitive skin. It's high in vitamin E and omega-3s like argan oil, but it's richer and goes on thicker, so it's terrific for rough, bumpy, or scaly skin. Similarly, **coconut oil** is full of omega-3 fatty acids, but it's a bit lighter than avocado oil. I recommend it for those with sensitive skin or who are prone to eczema. **Flaxseed oil** is rich in two kinds of fatty acids and works wonders on eczema and dermatitis. Other plant-based oils I love include borage seed, safflower, apricot kernel, olive, rose hip seed, neroli, and cranberry seed oil.

The wonderful thing about facial oils is that they are often inexpensive. I buy flaxseed oil and olive oil from the grocery store, in fact! Just be sure that whatever you buy is cold-pressed (heat destroys many beneficial molecular compounds) and organic (who wants pesticides on their skin?). You should also be aware that facial oil shouldn't be the only moisturizer you use. Oils are terrific at hydrating, but they're not good at replenishing like products with peptides or retinols are. While you can enjoy them as part of a serum or on their own under a heavier moisturizer, you should always back them up with a moisturizer that contains other, more complex ingredients.

oils i love

Indie Lee Squalane Facial Oil: Squalane is a stable form of squalene, a naturally occurring oil found in many plants, like olives, and I love it so much that I have it in one of my own serums! This facial oil is super lightweight, so no one has to fear being shiny or feeling oily under their makeup. It's loaded with antioxidants and makes me feel so hydrated!

Natura Bissé Diamond Extreme Oil: This oil is a bit of a splurge, but I love it because it focuses on all the right stuff, especially hydration and soothing dry skin that has become sensitized. It contains chia, amaranth, and calendula oils, as well as an omega-5 fatty acid.

My Rejuvenating Serum is a combination of oils, including olive oil, which reduces inflammation; rose hip oil, which increases circulation; jojoba oil, which balances sebum production; and argan oil, which protects elasticity. It won't clog your pores, so it's great even for people who break out.

RETINOLS

In the beauty industry, there is no substance more Googled, debated, praised, and misunderstood than retinol. In my opinion, retinol works miracles for fine lines, wrinkles, and dark spots, but it's not without its risks. Understanding it is key to using it effectively, and when you do, it may become the most trusted product in your beauty arsenal.

Retinols are derivatives of vitamin A that get converted by skin enzymes into retinoic acid. Retinols are frequently confused with retinoids, which are present in products such as Retin-A. Retinoids are also vitamin A derivatives, but retinols have a lower percentage of retinoic acid than retinoids do. They're therefore available over the counter, while retinoids are only available by prescription. Because their percentage of retinoic acid is lower, retinols also work more slowly. Both, however, affect gene expression, boost collagen production, and stimulate cell metabolism.

Retinol became an integral part of the beauty industry by accident. When it was first approved as an acne treatment in 1971, it was just that: a way to help people with moderate to severe cases of acne, and it was only available by prescription. But almost immediately, dermatologists noticed that it did more than just clear up pimples. They saw that their patients had dramatically smoother skin, fewer wrinkles and fine lines, and more even skin tone. Soon, the beauty industry jumped on it, and retinol became available over the counter in creams and serums.

When we start to age, cells don't regenerate as quickly as they did when we were young. Retinol directly affects gene expression, regulating that age-related issue by eliminating dead, dark skin cells and allowing fresh, new skin cells to come to the surface. Essentially, it goes deep into the layers of the skin, exfoliating, cleaning, and clearing as it soaks. It also clears up pimples because it cleans up the pores and eliminates bacterial growth.

Unfortunately, retinol's not without its downsides. Because it penetrates skin cells so deeply, it can cause redness, flakiness, dryness, and a high level of sensitivity. Some people who've used too much retinol look shiny, tight, and almost robotic. Some studies, including one from 2006 in the *International Journal of Environmental Research and Public Health*, suggest that retinol increases your skin's susceptibility to ultraviolet light, which could make you more likely to develop skin cancer. Therefore, I recommend using retinol only at night.

Because retinol can cause sensitivity, I suggest using retinol products that also contain a soothing agent, like fatty acids, chamomile, aloe, or green tea extract. In addition, recent technological advances have made it possible to fuse together the molecules in retinol, making it less harmful. There's also a new ingredient on the market called bakuchiol, a plant extract that penetrates deep into the layers of the cells just like retinol and delivers many of the same benefits but with fewer side effects.

If you have sensitive skin or haven't used retinol before, I recommend starting with a low concentration, like .025%. If you have problem-free skin that isn't easily irritated, you can try

glow from within

.25% at first, and if you're an old pro who's used retinol for years, you may level out at 1%. Use 2% or higher if you have a prescription or if you have a tremendous amount of sun damage, deep wrinkles, dark spots, or bad acne. Some skincare lines even go up to 5%, and this may be just fine for you. Simply experiment with what works on your skin.

People of any age can make retinol part of their skincare routine, and I urge women in their teens and twenties to try it, because there's no harm in slowing the effects of aging. It's simple to use, too. Just apply a pea-size amount of a retinol-based cream or serum to your face and neck. You can use it on wet, damp, or dry skin, but don't apply it over moisturizer. Try it twice a week at first, and if you don't have a reaction to it, you can up your usage to every other night, then nightly. In order to experience the deepest level of skin penetration, you might want to use it after you exfoliate, so your skin is especially smooth and receptive to it. Just bear in mind that retinol won't work immediately; it may take up to twelve weeks to produce noticeable results. Finally, because retinol affects gene expression and has been shown in some animal studies to affect pregnancy, pregnant women shouldn't use it.

●   ●   ●

retinol products i love

Jordan Samuel Skin Retinol Treatment Oil: This is a wonderful retinol treatment. Jordan's company is direct-to-consumer, so his pricing is very reasonable, but anyone in the beauty industry will tell you his formulas are spot-on. This product contains marula oil (from the nut of the marula tree) and cranberry seed oil to balance out the drying effects of vitamin A.

Renée Rouleau Advanced Resurfacing Serum: This serum is great for repairing sun damage or reversing the effects of aging on sensitive skin. It's balanced with peptides and glucosamine for super hydration, so it won't dry out your skin. I love the way this woman makes a formula, and you won't be disappointed!

My **Supernova Serum** is the formula I am most proud of, and it was voted Readers' Choice Best Serum by *InStyle* magazine in 2018. It combines vitamin A, chamomile, and fatty acids to soothe, balance, and hydrate, and retinol to promote rapid cell turnover and reveal younger-looking skin.

• • •

glow from within

TONERS

Anyone who grew up in the '80s and '90s remembers what toners used to be: alcohol-based to the extreme, they practically sucked the oil out of you the second you wiped them over your skin, leaving you tight and parched. Gone are those days, thank goodness, and now I consider toner to be a very useful part of a good beauty routine.

Toners should be used after you've removed your makeup and cleansed your skin. Unlike a face wash, there is no need to rinse off a toner; your skin will absorb it right away. Applied with a cotton pad or clean fingertips, the toner sweeps away any leftover residue, creating a fresh palette onto which you can apply serum, moisturizer, or other products. But depending on their ingredients, toners can be much more than just an extra step in cleansing, offering benefits like soothing, clarifying, and moisturizing your skin, while also restoring its pH balance.

The type of toner you should use is entirely dependent on your skin type. While people with very dry skin don't need to use toner, I believe it is a must if you have oily skin. If you have acne, I recommend using a toner that contains salicylic acid. If your skin is sensitive, choose one that contains calming ingredients, like calendula or other plant botanicals. People with dull skin may prefer a toner that contains a natural exfoliant, like papaya extract or lactic acid, while aging skin usually responds well to toners with hyaluronic acid or rose water. Trust me, there are hundreds and hundreds of toners on the market for almost all types of skin, and you can find one that's best for you just by reading the label, checking out reviews online, and trying them out.

If you have oily skin, apply toner as often as twice a day after cleansing. If you have dry skin, you should look for a nourishing, hydrating rose water spray or some other type of hydrating formula. After applying toner, always remember to moisturize within a minute so that your skin can hydrate immediately.

toners i love

Eminence Organic Skin Care toners: This company makes great toning sprays for all skin types. My favorites include the Sweet Red Rose Tonique for normal skin, the Wild Plum Tonique for dry skin, and the Neroli Age Corrective Hydrating Mist for hydrating aging skin.

four

YOUR

SELF-CARE

ROUTINE

The most radiant, healthy-looking men and women I see in my salon every day are those who've mastered the art of self-care. Sure, it helps that they choose the right products and treatments and don't eat foods that are bad for them, but they've also come to understand that being kind to themselves is as essential to the health of their skin as moisterizing, exfoliating, and eating lots of greens. They pay attention to their bodies, get plenty of sleep, work on reducing stress, exercise, and make time for connection and joy. They know that if you're stressed, exhausted, or sick all the time, or have developed bad habits like staying up late, smoking, or not wearing sunscreen, you're not only abusing yourself, you're abusing your skin.

That's why, when I meet with clients, I spend as much time talking to them about their lifestyles and habits as I do giving them facials. If a stressed-out, work-till-the-wee-hours corporate attorney comes to me begging for help getting rid of the dark circles under her eyes, I need her to understand that no magic facial is going to make her glow from within. She needs more restorative sleep, the proper amount of exercise, and a healthy way to process her stress. I'm a working mom of two, so I know how impossible it can be to get to the gym every day or develop a consistent yoga practice, but I want my clients to understand how even just the tiniest bit of self-care can make a world of difference for their skin. We *all* want to look good, and the truth is that when our bodies feel healthy, we look healthy. So treat your body, mind, and spirit as well as you treat your skin, because even the smallest amount of neglect is going to show all over your face.

•   •   •

healthy habits to boost your glow

EXERCISE

I'm sure you're aware that regular exercise is vital for your health and well-being—both in the short term and as you grow older. But did you know that exercise can also improve the appearance of your skin? That's right—the science is clear: moderate to strenuous exercise done a few times a week can benefit your skin all the way down to the cellular level.

Around age forty, the stratum corneum (the outer layer of the epidermis that's made up mostly of dead skin cells) starts to thicken. When this happens, your skin begins to look tough, and can take on a leathery appearance. At the same time, the dermis, which is right under the epidermis, starts to thin out, making your skin look hollow and saggy.

In 2011, researchers from McMaster University in Ontario released a study reporting that regular exercise—even if it's started late in life—can reverse this pattern, allowing the stratum corneum to thin while the dermis thickens. It was a remarkable finding that got a lot of attention, and for good reason! Led by weapon is boxing. She boxes four times a week and leads an extremely healthy, active lifestyle.

A few years ago, I lost a close friend to cancer, and the grief was unbearable. I stopped taking care of myself, until Helena stepped in and gave me the best present anyone could have given me: a month of sessions with her boxing trainer, Jason. It changed my life. Regular exercise has improved my health in so many ways: my mood has improved, I have more energy, I'm at a healthier weight, and, as a big bonus, client after client has told me I look younger!

Anyone who's ever been active can tell you that even though a good workout can be tough, after it's over, you immediately feel more vibrant and alive. Over time, exercise makes you stronger, boosts your outlook, and, according to recent research, improves your sleep quality by up to 65 percent.

How much exercise is enough? As a general guideline, you should aim to reach 40 to 60 percent of your maximum heart rate (which is 220 minus your age) three to five times a week. Our muscle mass decreases by 1 percent each year starting at age thirty, so it's best to intersperse cardiovascular exercise with strength training. Just be aware that when it comes to getting your heart pounding, you can do too much of a good thing. A 2008 study published in *Free Radical Biology and Medicine* showed that very high levels of strenuous exercise—near your maximum heart rate for the duration of your workout—can cause an increase of free radicals in your bloodstream. However, you can combat the effects of free radicals by eating a diet that's rich in antioxidants.

Because your blood vessels dilate during exercise, allowing them to release heat, a hard workout may also aggravate skin conditions like rosacea. But that's an easy problem to fix. Simply keep a cool cloth near you while you work out and place it on your face when you start to feel flushed. If you're outside running or cycling, splash some water from your water bottle on your face from time to time. Finally, a lot of people worry that sweating excessively may lead to acne, but that's not entirely true. Sweat is sterile, and you'll only develop problems if you let it accumulate and clog your pores. So always be sure to wash your face—and the rest of your body—after a tough workout.

STRESS MANAGEMENT

I'm sure this comes as no surprise to any of you, but stress is bad for you. It can lead to everything from headaches to heart problems to diabetes, and it can wreak havoc on your complexion. Existing conditions like psoriasis and eczema might worsen, or new problems like acne or dry, flaky skin may crop up. That's why stress management is such an important healthy habit to maintain—for your skin, your health, *and* your sanity.

Stress is a natural reaction to unforeseen events, and the fight-or-flight reaction produced by the flood of hormones from your adrenal glands during times of stress may save your life. Just ask anyone who's reflexively slammed on the brakes to avoid a car accident, or who's sprinted home during a sudden thunderstorm. But when stress is particularly intense or constant—as is the case in our society today, where we're flooded with a 24/7 news cycle, balancing work and life demands, dealing with the responsibilities of having a family, and more—it may lead to psychological or behavioral issues. Overtaxed, overworked people frequently experience sleeplessness, drink too much, pick at their skin or nails, eat too much sugar, drink too much coffee, or don't exercise enough. All these bad habits affect your skin.

The way stress operates inside your body is straightforward. When we perceive something threatening, our adrenal glands produce cortisol and adrenaline, two hormones that signal us to run, attack, or protect ourselves. These hormones cause our heart to race, our hairs to stand up, and our bodies to tense. But they also signal our sebaceous glands to produce more oil. Too much sebum may then lead to clogged pores, blackheads, pimples here and there, or a bad case of acne.

When cortisol levels increase, blood sugar levels also rise. Over time, this can lead to diabetes, but in the short term, it encourages glycation, the process that binds sugar and protein in our bodies, to happen within our skin. Glycation hardens your collagen, causing it to break down, which in turn can lead to fine lines and wrinkles.

Cortisol also decreases the production of hyaluronic acid, the substance that helps your skin cells hold in water and maintains its hydration levels. Less hyaluronic acid can mean dry patches, scaly or flaky skin, or an outbreak of psoriasis, rosacea, or eczema. Rising levels of cortisol also cause inflammation, a natural bodily defense against foreign threats like pollutants or viruses. But when there's no actual battle to fight—just a perceived one—inflammation can lead to acne.

The skin is one of the last parts of the body reached by the circulatory system, so when you're under stress, adrenaline signals your body to conserve blood flow. Your body thinks you're in danger, so it saves the blood for the heart, lungs, digestive system, or any other part of your body that needs energy to fight or escape. With less blood flowing to the surface of your skin, your skin cells don't receive enough oxygen or nutrients. This causes them to be unable to regenerate, and they die, leaving you with dull, lifeless skin.

Reducing stress in your life is easier said than done, much of the time, but I'm firmly of the opinion that if you add even one or two stress-relieving activities to your life every day, you're going to feel (and look!) much better. For me, those practices include exercise and a relaxing, mindful activity. I wake up two hours before my kids do so I can have some much-needed me time, and I usually read a book or ride my Peloton bike before I get them up for school. Those two activities relieve my stress *immediately*, and they've made a world of difference in my life. You can really do anything that makes you feel good, including yoga, running, walking, painting, knitting, or even hugging your husband, kids, or dog. I promise you that a little bit of human (or canine!) love will make your life less stressful. I also recommend taking supplements like vitamin C, which helps boost your immune system and regulates cortisol levels, and vitamin B, which alleviates nervousness and anxiety.

In a study conducted by Nobel Prize–winning scientist Elizabeth Blackburn, research subjects who implemented a mindfulness practice in their lives showed, after four to six months, a 30 percent increase in telomerase, the enzyme that impacts the length of a chromosome's telomeres (the protective caps at the ends of a strand of DNA). Longer telomeres have been proven to be associated with longevity, so it follows that practicing yoga, meditating, or journaling may help slow the aging process.

SLEEP

We've all heard the term "beauty sleep," but many of my clients don't fully understand how accurate it is. Getting an adequate amount of restorative sleep on a nightly basis is an essential part of your long-term health *and* your beauty routine.

So many of us are overstressed and overscheduled, frazzled and pulled in so many directions that the idea of getting a good night's sleep is—apologies for the terrible pun—something we can only dream of. In a recent survey, almost 25 percent of Americans said they were so tired that they often couldn't concentrate during the day. Another 11.3 percent reported that a lack of sleep had recently interfered with their ability to drive safely, and 8.6 percent said that not sleeping enough has affected their job performance. Lack of sleep is such an issue in our society that the Centers for Disease Control have declared it a public health epidemic!

But what qualifies as a "good night's sleep"? The National

decrease overnight, too. Cortisol breaks down collagen and elastin, and persistently high cortisol levels can lead to acne breakouts. Finally, the skin produces more antioxidants during sleep, and antioxidants are key to fighting environmental damage from free radicals.

I remember the first time I met my client Gwendoline Christie, a star of *Game of Thrones*. She greeted me with such genuine joy that I was bowled over. To this day, she is one of the happiest, most positive, funniest people I have ever known, with the heart of a true artist in every way. But a few years back, she was in New York to attend fashion week, as well as to shoot another project. This woman, whose endless energy cannot be stopped, had finally reached her limit. She was *exhausted*, and her always-perfect skin looked tired, just like the rest of her. Its color was dull, and while she wasn't broken out, her skin texture wasn't its usual silky soft.

I decided to do a fruit acid peel followed by LED light therapy, and her skin instantly woke back up. Instead of talking a mile a minute like we usually do during treatments, I let her sleep, and when she woke up, I finished with a session of microcurrent therapy. The peel got rid of the buildup of dead skin cells and surface dirt from too many airplane rides, the light calmed down the redness from the peel, and the microcurrent stimulated her lymphatic system. The damage wrought by lack of sleep had undone her, but after her facial, she looked eighteen again. Obviously, a good facial isn't a substitute for sleep, but it was the best I could do, and I think it truly helped Gwendoline.

What can you do to get more sleep—and thus look better in the morning—other than to go to bed earlier? First off, don't drink alcohol within ninety minutes of going to bed. Alcohol inhibits REM sleep, which is the time when your skin cells regenerate, and it's been proven that as few as two servings of alcohol right before bed will disrupt REM sleep throughout the night. Second, turn off all screens within ninety minutes of lights out. Whatever you're watching or whatever work crisis you're attempting to solve not only stimulates your brain, but the blue-spectrum light emitted by the TV or computer screen is identical to the rays of the sun, so it impacts your melatonin levels. This wakes you up. If you struggle to fall asleep within fifteen minutes of going to bed, get up and go into another room where you can read or meditate. (If you stay in bed, you may subconsciously associate your bed with insomnia, and that will keep you up.)

Finally, the products you choose for bedtime may affect how you look when you wake up. Rough, low-thread-count sheets stick to your skin, so when you move around at night, you may pull your skin, which leads to wrinkles. If you don't have the budget for a higher thread count, try using a satin pillowcase. Not only is it super soft, but your skin will never stick to it (it also helps preserve a blow out!). I also love sleep masks because they help me sleep like a baby; if you wear one, just be sure it's not too tight on your face. Try switching the side of your body you sleep on as well; people who consistently sleep on one side tend to have more wrinkles on that side of their face, while people who sleep on their stomachs tend to have puffiness from fluid pooling around their eyes.

Sweet dreams!

ATTITUDE

I work with beautiful women every day, and I can tell you one thing for certain: their good genes and ability to choose and afford the best possible products and treatments are not the only factors that make them gorgeous. Their attractiveness lies in who they fundamentally are, how they feel about themselves, and how they treat others. Beauty is *not* skin deep. Your attitude and actions are written in every line on your face.

I have a young daughter, and her presence in my life has been one of the most rewarding experiences I could ever imagine. Yet day in and day out, I see the kinds of challenges she and her friends face. They see airbrushed images of women on Instagram and in beauty magazines, and they worry that they're not pretty enough or, worse, not good enough. I'm in the beauty industry, so I can't avoid these images. And I like looking at them! I *want* to make my clients look as healthy, glowing, and ageless as the woman on the cover of *Cosmo* or *Glamour.* However, I never forget that all that seemingly flawless, effortless beauty is, in part, smoke and mirrors. It's a curated reality, and you can't let it define you or your self-worth.

Research backs up the fact that true beauty comes from within. In 2016, the skincare company Olay studied 2,500 women and found 10 percent of them to be "exceptional agers." What does that mean? According to criteria Olay had defined, these 250 women looked up to ten years younger than their actual ages. When their biochemistry was studied closely, the scientists discovered that a full 80 percent of their skin-specific genes operated more efficiently because of several external factors, the most important of which were the time they'd spent sunbathing, whether they wore sunscreen every day, and their level of positivity. On an almost uniform level, the women who'd aged best said they had a healthy, optimistic outlook about their lives and who they were.

The connection between a good outlook and healthy skin was confirmed in another small-scale study as well. Recently,

LA physician and antiaging expert Howard Murad asked forty women to read a set of positive self-affirmations and write in a journal daily. After four weeks, he noted that all the women had higher levels of skin hydration and lower blood pressure. What do these two factors lead to? Younger, healthier skin.

Maintaining strong human connections is another way to boost your mental health. I work in a salon full of amazing women, and I can't tell you how happy my colleagues make me. These strong, smart ladies continually encourage and inspire me. Being in the company of these women sustains me and helps me stay positive even when work is stressful. All of us know this to be true anecdotally, but believe it or not, research has found that friendship can actually be lifesaving. One study that tracked women with early-stage breast cancer found that those who had strong friendships had a four times greater chance of survival than those who lacked such a network.

So, please, remember that beauty isn't found in the mirror, an Instagram post, or a jar. True beauty is the action you take in your life, the friends you make, and how you express yourself. Love yourself and others; it will make you *and* the world more beautiful.

● ● ●

bad habits that dim your glow

NERVOUS TICS AND OTHER PROBLEM BEHAVIORS

We all have our bad habits, but some are worse for our skin than others. In particular, there are ways we abuse our skin that are so subtle—or so rarely talked about—that we may not even realize we're doing lasting damage when we engage in them.

One of these imperceptible yet nasty habits is **face touching**. You may have a dry patch on your nose that you're desperate to scrape off, or perhaps you rest your cheeks in your hands when you're tired or bored. I bet that you didn't wash your hands right before doing either of these things, right? I didn't think so. When you touch your face without first washing your hands, you transfer dirt, chemicals, debris, and bacteria from your fingers and hands onto your face. These nasty foreign substances can clog your pores and lead to irritation and breakouts.

A lot of people **rub their eyes**, especially first thing in the morning after waking up. The area under the eyes is the thinnest, most sensitive skin on your whole face, so when you pull at it, you damage its elasticity. You may also break the tiny capil-laries just under the surface of the skin, which will cause purple undereye bags, or "raccoon eyes" as they're sometimes called.

Chewing gum isn't in and of itself a bad habit, but if you do it regularly, you're putting a lot of strain on the muscles of your jaw. These incredibly strong muscles already perform a lot of jobs, so this added repetitive motion stresses the face more, eventually breaking down collagen in the skin tissue, which leads to fine lines and wrinkles. Regularly **drinking through a straw** causes a similar problem with the muscles around your mouth, result-ing in fine lines above your upper lip.

Some of you out there might be chronic cheek biters. People who **bite the inside of their mouths** typically do so because of anxiety, so whatever they can do to help alleviate that stress may go a long way toward helping them stop. But from a purely cos-metic perspective, this bad habit makes your face look squished up and may lead to wrinkles and fine lines, especially on your upper lip and at the sides of your mouth.

Finally, a word about **cell phones**! Since many of us are positively glued to our mobile devices, I should warn you that they're absolutely *filthy*. A recent study revealed that 92 percent of phones are covered in bacteria, and *E. coli* is present on 16 percent. What's *E. coli*? It's a bacteria found in feces, and if ingested, it can make you really, really sick. Few of us wash our hands after checking our emails, so the likelihood that you're transferring *E. coli* from your phone to your fingers to your face is high. Please, sanitize your phone, or better yet, if you make or take calls frequently, invest in a hands-free device that will prevent you from ever having to put your phone close to your beautiful face.

SMOKING

This bad habit is so nasty, it deserves its own category. If you smoke, I don't think I'm telling you anything you haven't heard a million times already: hands down, smoking is one of the worst things you can do for your health. It also dramatically changes the way you look, harming your skin from both the inside and the outside. I know quitting is *so* hard, but trust me—if you do, you'll look years younger within a month. I've seen it happen!

I once had a friend of a friend who bought her mom a birthday facial with me. It was in the early days of my salon, so I was thrilled to be seeing a new client. When she lay down on the table, she told me two things: she had never had a facial before, and she was a frequent smoker. My original plan was to give her something antiaging, but after one look at her skin I realized I had to do an old-fashioned cleanse. Her pores were the size of saucers, and they were *full* of sebum. She had so many huge blackheads that I'm pretty sure she thought some of them were moles. They were the result of years of tar, dirt, smoke, and chemicals wafting across her nose, mouth, forehead, and cheeks; landing on her skin, and filling up her pores. Even though she washed her face regularly, it wasn't enough, and she needed my help. I can't swear that it was the most relaxing facial I've ever given, but I felt better knowing she left that day with her skin breathing easier and healthier as a result.

When you smoke, you also purse your lips and squint, so over time, fine lines begin to develop on your upper lip, the sides of your mouth, and around your eyes, making you look as if you're constantly puckering up. The damage is more than skin deep, though. The four thousand chemicals in cigarette smoke—fifty of which are carcinogenic—constrict blood flow throughout your body, including to the entire surface of your skin. In particular, nicotine decreases the microcirculation within the small blood vessels at the surface of the skin, which is why heavy smokers have a characteristic gray pallor. They're literally turning gray! It's estimated that for each cigarette you smoke, blood flow decreases for about thirty minutes, so if you smoke a pack of cigarettes a day, you are depriving your body of oxygen almost continuously during your waking hours. When blood flow is lessened, your skin doesn't get the nutrients it needs. Smoking helps unleash free radicals within the body, so antioxidants like vitamins C and E can't rise to the surface to fight them. Worse, the smoke even depletes the antioxidants, so you have fewer available to fight the free radicals in the first place.

The chemicals in cigarettes—particularly lipid peroxide—destroy collagen and elastin in the skin. This causes skin to become dry, withered, sallow, lifeless, and saggy. Without elastin, your cheeks lose their pillowy softness, increasing the puckered look. Further, fibroblasts, which are the cells that produce collagen, make 40 percent less collagen when they're exposed to cigarette smoke. This is true especially around the eye area, so smokers often have large dark circles under their eyes.

There's more! Cigarette smoke amplifies UV light as it touches the skin, so smoking increases your risk of skin cancer, particularly squamous cell carcinoma. Many people are surprised to hear this, since they assume that lung cancer is the major cancer risk from smoking, but some studies say that smoking puts you at an even greater risk of skin cancer than sunbathing!

Unfortunately, a smoker's skin doesn't respond well to treatment by an aesthetician. I can squeeze your blackheads all day, but you'll still have tar in your pores. I can give you LED light therapy to increase your collagen, but your compromised fibroblasts just won't make more collagen. If you stop smoking, however, your skin will get better. Your circulation returns to near normal almost immediately after your last cigarette, letting much-needed antioxidants do their job and allowing the gray pallor to disappear. Within twenty-eight days of quitting, your skin cells start to turn over, so old, dead cells make way for new collagen- and elastin-producing fibroblasts. With a little help from good products and an aesthetician, the plumpness will return, fine lines will diminish, and your skin will become hydrated again.

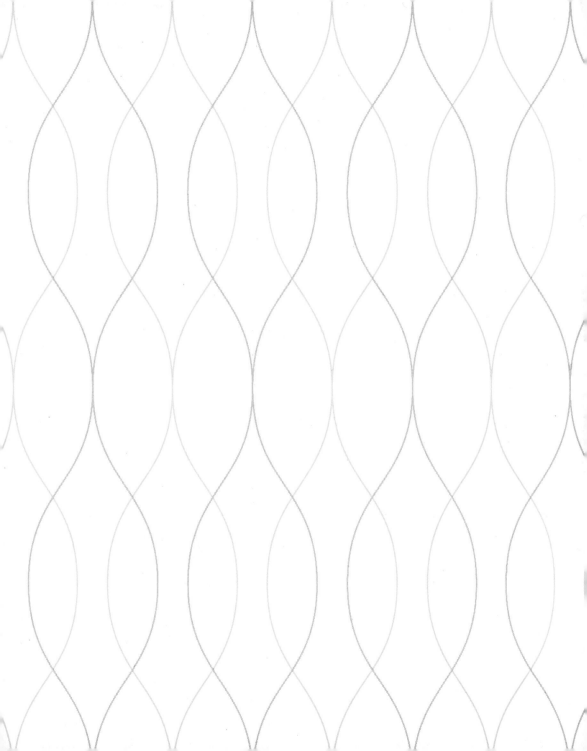

five

YOUR

SPA

ROUTINE

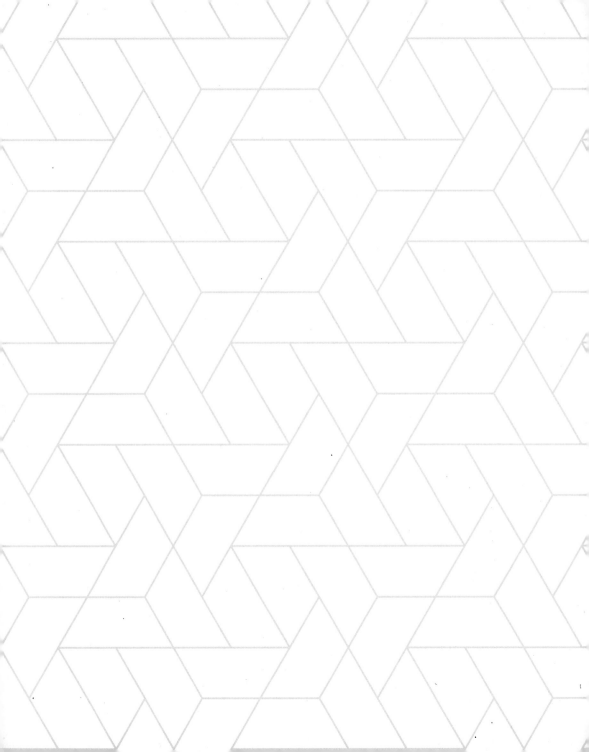

Maybe you're eating nutritious foods, Drinking plenty of water, getting your beauty sleep, and sticking to your skincare routine morning and night. Or maybe just the opposite is true— you've been working late, subsisting on takeout, and drinking a pot of coffee daily, and you can't remember the last time you exfoliated or even took off your makeup before bed. Whether you have your self-care routine down to a science or you're in desperate need of some TLC . . . a trip to the spa may be just the thing you need. Sure, giving facials is my job, so I'm biased, but I'm convinced that getting regular facials can take your skin to the next level *and* help to erase years from your face.

What does a facialist do that you can't do for yourself? First, a seasoned aesthetician can provide expert advice tailored to your skin condition(s), skin type, and lifestyle. You'll learn what you're already doing right and what you could do better, and you can take that knowledge home with you, implementing it in a routine that works best for you. Second, a good facial will unclog your pores and exfoliate your skin, and that allows your products to really penetrate and work more effectively. The hour you spend in a spa is also restorative, not just for your mind, but for your lymphatic system as well. When an aesthetician massages your face, neck, and head, your skin benefits from the improved circulation of blood and lymph, and may release toxins as well as excess water.

I know facials can be expensive. You might spend sixty dollars at some spas—even for just a half hour—or hundreds of dollars at others. I understand that you can only do what your budget allows, but I think women often underestimate the benefits of self-care. Your skin is a lifetime commitment. You came into this world wearing just your skin, and you'll leave with it on as well. It's worth it. *You* are worth it. So think hard about how you spend your money and carefully consider whether the occasional facial is for you.

If you do decide to schedule a facial, going every now and then—even once a year—can be hugely helpful for all the reasons I've mentioned. If you are able to make a spa visit a regular part of your routine, I recommend going about every six weeks. While you're there, you might get to experience some of the cool technology, scientific techniques, and specialized ingredients we'll cover in this chapter. With a better understanding of these interventions, you can walk into any aesthetician's office feeling calm and confident.

One final word about getting facials: I know it can feel embarrassing to see a facialist when your skin is acting up or at its worst, even though that may be when you need an aesthetician's help the most. Please know that your facialist has seen it all and is not judging you in any way! She is there to make your experience enjoyable, relaxing, and informative, and she can not only help to resolve the skin issues you're having, she can also help you put together a routine that will prevent you from having those problems in the future.

With that said, let's take a closer look at some of the most popular techniques being used in spas and clinics today.

•   •   •

specialty treatments

LASERS

When I tell people I'm an aesthetician, they often assume I spend my days scooping cream onto women's faces, steaming pores, and doing extractions. How wrong they are! My job requires me to keep up with the beauty industry's latest technology, much of which is downright fascinating. At the top of that exciting list are lasers.

Laser procedures are part of a larger category of light therapy. Lasers focus a beam of pulsating high-intensity light onto a specific area of the body. In short bursts, this light causes micro-injuries to the skin, resulting in collagen formation as the skin tries to heal itself and creating fresher, tighter-looking skin. This treatment is great for wrinkles and fine lines, acne scars, sagging skin, uneven pigmentation, age spots, mild to moderate sun damage, and more. Because it's an invasive treatment, laser procedures are given under local or topical anesthesia, with a full recovery time of about two weeks. This might sound like a long time, but trust me—the benefits are dramatic, and you'll notice more youthful, smoother skin almost immediately.

There are so many new lasers on the market right now that I'd have to write a whole separate volume on the subject. I get asked all the time which treatments are my favorites, so I'll share two that I recommend to every single one of my clients.

IPL stands for **intense pulsed light**, and it treats the skin using the full spectrum of light, as opposed to just one wavelength like other kinds of lasers use. IPL employs a process called photorejuvenation to address sun damage, uneven pigment, and dilated blood vessels. Although the treatment can be mildly painful and leave you swollen temporarily, it clears up pigment issues very successfully. But just to be clear, if you have sun damage, your cells have mutated, and just because your skin appears more even after this treatment doesn't mean your altered pigment has magically disappeared. That's why, after IPL, you have to be diligent about always wearing a hat and sunscreen, or the pigment will return.

Clear + Brilliant is a nonablative laser resurfacing treatment; "nonablative" means it doesn't heat and remove the top layer of the skin right away, but rather works much deeper over a short period of time. And work it does! I am absolutely *obsessed* with Clear + Brilliant. It stimulates collagen production, resurfaces, and evens out the pigment in the skin. You do need to be numbed in advance of the procedure, but nothing resurfaces and removes fine lines like this. The downtime is a few days of sunburn-level redness, but then your skin becomes hard, like sandpaper, as you shed that dead layer of skin. The results are really amazing, and you won't look like you've had work done. You'll just seem like a refreshed version of you!

LED LIGHT THERAPY

LED (light-emitting diode) light therapy has been getting a ton of press lately in beauty blogs and magazines. I think that's partly because everyone loves hearing about new, snazzy-sounding technology and can't wait to try it out, wondering if it really *does* hold the key to turning back the clock. I don't believe there's one magic button that will zap twenty years from your face, but I positively love LED light therapy. It's incredibly effective at fighting the symptons of aging, evening out skin tone, shrinking pore size, making your skin softer and more elastic, and helping it appear less coarse. It also reduces inflammation, makes the skin less reactive to environmental pressures, speeds healing of the body by as much as 300 percent, and clears up acne (because it kills bacteria).

Elisabeth Moss is one of my favorite people. She's funny as hell, beautiful, and kind to everyone. She is a true queen. I met her originally through her makeup artist Daniel Martin just as she was about to start all sorts of crazy press for the first season of *The Handmaid's Tale.* Elisabeth's skin is beautiful, but it's sensitive and reactive to everything. I wanted to make her glow, but it was a challenge because every touch made her red.

We did two LED light sessions during her first appointment, as well as a microcurrent facial, and afterward, Elisabeth was positively glowing—her skin looked lit from within. The next day I texted her and told her to buy an at-home LED light machine so she could use it often to try to build up her skin's strength. She did, and the results have been amazing.

I know you're probably wondering, *What exactly* is *LED light treatment? Does it involve some sort of weird tanning bed that's going to burn my eyeballs or give me skin cancer?* Not at all. LED light therapy doesn't utilize ultraviolet light, but rather red and near-infrared light, which are on a lower, gentler part of the electromagnetic spectrum. I find the science behind this technology fascinating. At the turn of the nineteenth century, researchers discovered that certain infrared light waves would stimulate energy in living cells, both plant and human. Almost a century later, in the late 1980s, NASA took this original study and developed technology called High Emissivity Aluminiferous Luminescent Substrate (HEALS) to help grow plants on space shuttle missions. NASA later realized that HEALS might have more practical healing applications, and they commissioned a company to create machines that only gave off certain light waves. Now light therapy is an FDA-approved therapy in cancer treatment, sports medicine, and—lucky for you—the beauty industry!

LED light therapy is used anytime during facials. A lightbulb that emits only red and near-infrared light is placed behind small panels, which are then positioned a few inches from your skin. As the light shines on you, it fuels the cells in your dermis, causing them to produce higher levels of collagen and elastin. Trust me, it works!

LED light therapy isn't used exclusively to treat the face. In fact, you may look wrinkle-free from the waist up, but have droopy, sagging skin on the rest of your body. To help combat this, I created and patented an LED light bed that I call "The Time Machine," which looks sort of like a tanning bed; I have one in each of my salons. The Time Machine uses red and near-infrared light (which I've found to be more effective than the amber or blue light emitted by other devices) to target areas like your butt, thighs, stomach—anywhere that needs a little pick-me-up.

I've seen dramatic results from the LED light bed. A few years ago, one of my longtime employees was bitten in the face by a dog. She called me right after she left the hospital with forty stitches in her face. Dreading the scar she knew would form soon, she begged me for help, and while I said I couldn't promise anything, I knew the science behind LED light therapy. I told her that after her stitches were removed, she should use the light bed in our office every day, without fail. She did. We took photos of her daily, and at the end of two weeks, she had no bruising and no scar.

The great news is that an LED light treatment with an aesthetician takes only about twenty minutes, and the results are almost immediate. After two or three treatments, the skin looks healthier, more elastic, plumper, and clearer.

MICROCURRENT THERAPY

I'm always on the lookout for new technologies, and it's amazing when I find one only to discover that it's not new at all, but has existed quietly under the radar for decades. That was the case with microcurrent therapy, a technology that's more than fifty years old.

Just after World War II, a surgeon named Dr. Carlos Matteucci, who was treating soldiers with bone fractures and bone implants, realized that his patients experienced better, faster overall healing if their muscles didn't atrophy. But many of these men were bedridden, so they were unable to get up and exercise; muscle atrophy was inevitable. The doctor thought about the problem and decided to try using a low-level electrical current to stimulate their muscles. Sure enough, his patients soon began to develop muscle tone, and they healed faster. The beauty industry caught wind of this discovery, jumped on it, and, by the 1960s, had integrated it into some salon and dermatological therapies. Today, I use microcurrent therapy daily in my most popular facials.

The face is made up of forty-three muscles. We use many of these—such as the muscles of the mouth—all the time. However, there are others we rarely use, and just like the muscles of those bedridden soldiers, they begin to atrophy, wither, and sag. Microcurrent technology employs tiny waves that mimic the electrical output of your cells. Using a pair of two-pronged handheld devices, I send these gentle waves of electricity through your skin, where they stimulate your cells and give your unused muscles a little workout—basically acting as a personal trainer for your face.

The results are almost immediate. Your facial muscles tighten ever so slightly, so there's a noticeable lifting of your skin. Your jawline may look more defined, your cheeks may plump up, making your cheekbones look more prominent, and one eyebrow may inch slightly higher than the other. This tautness makes you seem more alert and aware, as if you've just had a night of deep, restorative sleep.

Microcurrent therapy doesn't just work wonders on your muscles. It also drains water from your face, giving your lymphatic system a much-needed flush. As you age, the skin cells in your epidermis become less active, which is why they produce less collagen and elastin. Studies have shown that microcurrent therapy increases the production of collagen by up to 14 percent, elastin production by 48 percent, and blood circulation by 38 percent.

And that's not all! Adenosine triphosphate (ATP) is the molecule that holds all your body's energy for muscular and cellular function. But your body doesn't store ATP by placing it on reserve like it does with the fat in your fat cells. Instead, your cells manufacture it as needed. A study from the early 1980s showed that microcurrents increase levels of ATP by 500 percent. With more energy at the ready, your cells can work more efficiently and respond to cellular damage more quickly.

Microcurrent therapy is something I use on my clients on the morning of the Oscars every year. It takes the tiredness out of their eyes and makes their face look contoured, lifted, and tight—instantly. I remember one year, I was due to see an

Oscar-nominated actress whom I hadn't met before. You never know what to expect when you see a client for the first time, so I had to be ready for anything. She walked through the door, and I immediately knew something was wrong. She looked pale and puffy, and when I asked her if she was okay, she told me she'd spent the night throwing up from food poisoning. I had one hour to help her, so I decided to do a microcurrent facial and hope for the best. When I asked her to look in the mirror at the end, she couldn't believe her eyes. The microcurrent stimulation of her lymphatic system helped deliver fresh nutrients to her face while removing all the excess water that had made her look puffy and tired. Microcurrents had wiped away her bout of food poisoning and transformed her into the glamorous movie star she is.

I recommend that anyone—young or old—try microcurrent therapy and do it as often as their budget allows. The electrical flow from the wands is so low that it doesn't hurt one bit, and many of my clients report that they like the tingly, energizing feeling it gives them. As a bonus, the products you use at the end of the facial and in the days and weeks afterward penetrate your skin more deeply, helping you get that glow-from-within look more effortlessly than before.

MICRODERMABRASION

Microdermabrasion, an intense form of exfoliation that removes the top layer of dead skin from your face, hands, neck—or entire body, if you like—was invented in Italy in the late 1980s. Thirty years is *eons* in terms of technology within the skincare industry, so many people assume that, as far as treatments go, microderm-abrasion is now passé. I disagree. The techniques and ingredients used in this treatment have evolved and are gentler than they once were, and the results it can achieve are outstanding.

From the late 1980s through the '90s, microdermabrasion in-volved an aesthetician using a handheld wand to spray aluminum oxide crystals—the second-hardest crystal, after diamond—against a client's face. The procedure essentially blasted away the client's dead skin cells, which the facialist would vacuum up, along with the crystals, after finishing the microdermabrasion. When research linked aluminum oxide to a higher risk of developing cancer, aestheticians began taking steps to limit their exposure to it, and many switched to using sodium bicarbonate crystals. But those often proved too soft to effectively abrade the skin. Today, some people use corundum powder, but I prefer a process called diamond-tipped microdermabrasion, also known as a diamond peel. Sound fancy? It's actually quite simple.

Diamond peels are performed using a wand with an abrasive tip made of laser-cut diamonds. During the procedure, the facialist lightly presses the tip of the wand against the client's skin and moves it across the face to lightly loosen, then lift off the dead skin cells. As the device exfoliates, a small vacuum within the wand sucks up the dead skin cells. There's no mess of crystals flung out everywhere, just deep, gentle peeling. Typically, the whole process can take anywhere from five minutes to half an hour, and you see results immediately afterward. As with any exfoliation, your skin feels a bit smoother, but more than that, it's noticeably softer and more pliable, as if your skin has traveled a few years back in time. The results of a microdermabrasion typically last from a few days to a few weeks.

Microdermabrasion helps to diminish fine lines, gives you a glow, reduces enlarged pores, removes age spots, brightens your complexion, and can assist with hyperpigmentation. I've discovered that it can even help with acne scars, unless they're very deep (raw, red scars from a particularly bad case of acne should be treated with lasers).

Microdermabrasion also increases blood flow near the surface of the skin, which helps stimulate the growth of collagen. This, in turn, improves your skin's elasticity, which makes you look visibly younger. The products you use on your skin also become more effective right away because they can easily penetrate into the dermis, rather than having to soak through a layer of dead skin cells first.

Microdermabrasion has declined in popularity recently because there are so many new treatments available—especially noninvasive ones like chemical peels, oxygen therapy, and LED light therapy—that deliver longer-term results (meaning a few weeks to a few months). All these treatments are great, and I have few bad things to say about them, but microdermabrasion is a *classic* that gives immediate results. In fact, I like it so much that I include it as a complimentary treatment in all the facials offered at my salon. I do charge for microdermabrasion on the legs, arms, buttocks, or any other area that feels rough, but otherwise, facial microdermabrasion is a standard part of the treatment package I deliver.

There may be some immediate side effects after microdermabrasion, but they're not major and won't last long. Some people notice a bit of redness from burst capillaries, so if you have especially sensitive skin, you should tell your aesthetician before undergoing a treatment. People who are prone to breakouts or cold sores may notice irritation as well, but again, if this is the case for you, simply notify your facialist beforehand and he or she can tailor your session accordingly.

MICRONEEDLING

I know, I know. Any cosmetic treatment with the word "needle" in it probably makes shivers go up your spine. Never fear! Microneedling is a safe and relatively painless procedure that can deliver dramatic results to the most problematic skin—if it's done correctly.

Microneedling is a form of collagen-induction therapy (CIT) that uses short, narrow, densely packed needles to penetrate the epidermis and break up collagen bundles in the dermis. This causes collagen production in the epidermis to go into overdrive in an attempt to heal the superficial damage the needles have done to the skin. With abundant, active collagen hard at work, the skin starts to regenerate, becoming firmer, more radiant, and more lifted almost immediately. Dark circles under the eyes begin to fade, and wrinkles even out, giving the appearance of younger, healthier skin. Some people even report that their skin is almost pillowy, like they've regained some of the soft, plump baby fat they had when they were kids.

Microneedling is incredibly effective at reducing the appearance of acne scars, particularly atrophic scars, which are the differently sized and shaped indented scars that give acne-prone skin an uneven texture. In a 2015 study published in the *Journal of Clinical and Aesthetic Dermatology*, ten patients with significant scarring from acne were given six sessions of microneedling at two-week intervals over three months; afterward, their skin showed dramatic improvement. The depth of their scarring wasn't as profound, their redness had faded, and, overall, their skin texture looked more even.

Still, you're probably thinking, *But there are needles, and I hate needles!* I get it—no one likes needles, especially needles in close proximity to their face. Think of it like you would acupuncture. These needles are *tiny*—about 2.5 millimeters long and as thin or thinner than acupuncture needles. They're also spaced so close together that they deliver about three hundred tiny pricks per square inch of skin. This means you feel an overall pressure on your face rather than one massive jab. The needles can be mounted on a dermaroller (a rotating cylinder with a handle) or a dermastamp (a block attached to a handle), or couched in the tip of a Dermapen (a device that looks like a pen). I'm not a big fan of the dermaroller because it tends to leave path marks on the skin, so I use an FDA-approved machine that combines microneedling with radio frequency.

About thirty minutes to an hour before a microneedling

treatment, a dermatologist or aesthetician will put a numbing cream on your face and allow it to soak in and penetrate the layers of your skin. When your face is just slightly numb, the aesthetician will begin to move the microneedling device across your face, lightly brushing your skin in upward strokes and small circles. When the treatment is complete, I always apply hyaluronic acid, followed by an EGF facial mask, an LED light therapy session, and an oxygen treatment.

Most people report that any discomfort is very tolerable, like they're being lightly scratched. Sometimes, there's a bit of bleeding, but it's usually minimal and only in a few spots. Most people aren't bothered by it because their skin looks and feels so clean, soft, and fresh afterward. By the next day, my clients report that their products penetrate deeply, revealing skin that's noticeably plumper, more radiant, and positively glowing from within.

Within the last few years, at-home dermarollers have become incredibly popular, partly because they're so cheap, around $20 or less. I'm not in favor of microneedling at home for a few reasons. First, the needles on most nonprofessional dermarollers are only .2 to 1 millimeter long, which isn't enough to penetrate through the epidermis into the dermis. If you can't go deep enough, you can't break up collagen bundles, which means you're damaging your skin for no reason. Second, these needles aren't hygienic. No matter how much you wash them, they quickly become breeding grounds for bacteria and viruses, which, when you use the device, can enter and spread under the skin, causing infection. And in 2017, the FDA raised the idea of regulating dermarollers because of their potential to damage nerves and blood vessels and cause infections. These risks are unlikely if you see an aesthetician, who uses sterile equipment and is trained in the procedure.

For best results, I recommend microneedling three times a year, with at least four to six weeks between treatments. When performed by a professional, this fantastic treatment will make your skin look as good as new.

OXYGEN THERAPY

A few years ago, oxygen treatments were garnering huge, splashy headlines. Madonna told the press that she loved them so much, she bought oxygen therapy machines for every one of her houses—and I can only imagine how many houses she owns! The trend caught on, and before I owned my own salon, I worked in places that had oxygen tanks in all their treatment rooms.

Some critics were skeptical, saying there was little data to back up claims that oxygen helps your skin, but I do oxygen treatments after every facial in both of my salons, and I can promise you that I see massive results in *all* my clients.

Oxygen is one of the greatest life forces in the world. In hospitals, hyperbaric chambers, which are filled with 100% oxygen and pressurized, are used to help certain patients recover. When you exercise, your cells become oxygenated, which improves your overall metabolic function. Your skin is no different. If it gets enough oxygen, it functions better, increasing cell turnover and producing the collagen and elastin that help you look young. If it doesn't get enough oxygen, it withers, sags, and becomes dull.

So why wouldn't taking a brisk walk outdoors—where there's plenty of oxygen—improve the overall look and function of your skin? Our environment is highly polluted, so the air that's hitting your face is full of carbon monoxide, dirt, debris, and all kinds of toxins that wreak havoc on your skin. Oxygen treatment is more refined. It gives your skin a blast of 98 percent pure oxygen, without pollutants, and that helps your skin look plumper, firmer, and more lifted.

When I do oxygen treatments, I use a machine attached to a small, handheld wand. The tip of the wand delivers a spray of atomized serum through pressurized oxygen, so not only does your face receive the life-giving benefits of pure oxygen, but it's hydrated by a serum of hyaluronic acid, aloe, green tea extract, and vitamins A, E, and C. With more hydrated, plumper, oxygenated skin, products are absorbed more easily, and are therefore more effective. Because the air in an oxygen treatment is so pure, it also fights bacteria, toxins, and other pathogens that lie on your skin, which makes you look cleaner, healthier, and more radiant. Plus, oxygen just *feels* good. My clients report that they love the tingly feeling of the mist on their face, and they bask in the instant hydration they get from the serum.

Oxygen has become a very popular ingredient in many over-the-counter beauty products, especially creams and masks, so I'm often asked whether these products are as effective as an oxygen treatment. My answer is yes and no. While these products don't deliver the high concentration of pure oxygen that an oxygen facial will, people do report that over time, their skin looks firmer and more radiant. This makes sense to me; with more oxygen in your skin, you experience better circulation, and that will help your skin look and feel healthier.

• • •

LYMPHATIC DRAINAGE MASSAGE

Lymphatic massage is one of my favorite ways to help reduce puffiness, eliminate dark circles under the eyes, and lessen the frequency of breakouts. Most facialists will give you a lymphatic massage as a part of your facial, but you don't have to go to the spa to benefit from this therapy—you can do it yourself at home.

Your lymphatic system relies on good nutrition, plenty of water, and exercise to keep lymph moving. When you're under the weather, not eating right, or sedentary, your lymphatic system slows down, and that's when impurities and fluids pool beneath the surface of your skin.

Lymphatic massage isn't just the fancy work of aestheticians like me; it's rooted in ninety years of science. In the 1930s, a group of Danish doctors practicing in Cannes, France, discovered that massaging their patients' lymph nodes helped them recover from their illnesses faster—and made their skin more radiant. Over the years, this simple massage practice became known as "French touch," because French women loved doing it at home. Unfortunately, it's become a lost art in the United States, and a lot of women who get regular facials don't even realize their aestheticians are doing it.

glow from within

I recommend lymphatic massage for anyone—whether your skin is dry, oily, or combination. It is so easy to do, and best of all, it takes less than ten minutes; you can do it in the morning or evening, as often as you like. Here's how:

Start with clean, dry skin, and position your index and middle fingers just underneath your ears, in the soft indentation behind your jawbone. Using gentle but firm pressure, rub your fingers down, then loop back in a "J" motion. Don't just graze the surface of your skin, but don't crush your lymphatic tubes, either. Continue this "J" pattern three times, then move to the middle of your neck, right on the sides near your arteries. Do the same at the base of your neck, about an inch above your clavicles. Finally, move to where your neck meets your collarbone and massage the soft part along the same neck line you've been following.

It's time to move to your chin. Using your pointer, middle, and ring fingers, massage in the "J" pattern three times on your chin, below your lips but to the right and left of your chin cleft. Shift your fingers along your jawline, below the corners of your lips, and rub there. Then go to the far end of your jawline, to the muscles where many of us hold tension.

Using the two fingers you started with, go back to your first position, under your ears, and massage there. Move down your neck in a line, working the same positions you pressed on your neck previously. Then go under your eyes, massaging in the "J" pattern along your eye orbit, from the sides of your nose to just below the outer corners of your eyes. End at the place where your cheekbones meet the sides of your eyes. If you've got puffy eyes, especially in the morning, this will dramatically improve undereye bags.

Where does the fluid from your puffy eyes drain? Down the sides of your face. To move that excess liquid through your lymphatic vessels, massage the sides of your face, right toward the top of your ears, then shift down to the middle of your ears, then to the bottom of your ears, where your jawline begins. Finally, return to your neck, right where you began, and travel the length of your neck once again.

Now reposition your fingers on your forehead, right above your eyebrows. Rub three times here, then move along your forehead, massaging in the middle, and finish at your temples. If you're prone to breakouts on your forehead, this will help clear out the inflammation that triggers them. Because the fluid needs to drain, move to your ear position and massage there, then finish up along you neck. It's vital you remember your neck, because this is where the excess liquid eventually drains out into your tissues.

That's it! I find lymphatic massage so soothing, yet invigorating, and I consider it a part of my daily routine. It gives my skin a much-needed boost, and it makes me feel great.

PEELS

A lot of people are hesitant about doing a peel. Most of my clients assume they are dangerous and have heard at least one horror story about a peel gone wrong (or maybe they just can't forget that episode of *Sex and the City*, where Samantha attended Carrie's book launch party after a supposed "quickie lunchtime peel," with her face so red, it looked like a piece of raw beef). The truth is that peels get a bad rap, and most of the time, they are perfectly safe.

Peels are just an extreme form of exfoliation. They help dissolve or slough away dead skin cells, allowing the skin to regenerate and become brighter, clearer, and more radiant. Peels can help stimulate collagen production, clear discoloration, eliminate fine lines and rough red patches, and give the skin a more youthful appearance. But when it comes to choosing the right peel, you need to carefully consider the needs of your skin and how it might respond to the treatment. In order to do that, it's important to understand the differences among the types of peels available at spas and in your dermatologist's office.

Chemical peels are probably the most well-known—and most feared—type of peels. When I started out as an aesthetician in the '90s, these were *all* the rage, and my clients were positively shocked that any other treatment could give them the dramatic results they were looking for. Today, I don't perform chemical peels in my spas, but not because I don't think they are useful. Quite the opposite—I think they can give great results if done properly.

Chemical peels involve putting some form of acid, which hasn't been mixed with another cosmetic ingredient, directly on the skin and allowing it to penetrate the dermatologic layers and dissolve dead skin cells. The acid literally burns away some of the skin, and this damage causes new skin to form. A mild peel—the aforementioned "lunchtime peel"—is usually done with a gentle alpha hydroxy acid like lactic or salicylic acid, which penetrates the epidermis but doesn't go deeply into the dermis. After a mild peel, it takes one to seven days for the skin to heal completely, and you may be slightly red or have scaly skin for at least a day.

You do need to wear extra moisturizer and sunscreen for a week after the treatment, but you can put on makeup the next day.

Moderate peels typically use glycolic acid, which penetrates the dermis. They're often used to treat more severely damaged, discolored, or aging skin, and they can successfully eliminate precancerous lesions like actinic keratoses. The recovery time is longer—about one to two weeks—and the side effects are greater. You may have blisters, swollen eyelids, or very red, patchy skin.

Chemical peels are intense the deeper they go, and that's why you should never have one if you've recently used a product containing retinol or vitamin C, both of which can be irritating. You also have to be careful not to book peels too regularly, as they can break down the stratum corneum, the layer responsible for protecting the skin from bacteria and viruses, and possibly leave it inflamed. Chemical peels also cause your skin to become very sensitive and dry, so you must stay out of direct sun for days to weeks, liberally apply sunscreen, and moisturize more than you normally would. All that said, when the results are in, they can be astounding!

Because I'm not a dermatologist, I tend to use natural ingredients for gentler peels. I prefer **fruit enzyme peels**, which are milder than even lactic acid peels. In this type of peel, the enzymes from fruits like pumpkin, pineapple, papaya, kiwi, cherry, orange, and mango are combined with alpha lipid acid, coenzyme Q10, antioxidants, vitamins, and something that helps circulation, like neroli oil. This mixture breaks up keratin, a protein in the dermis, then dissolves and removes dead surface cells. The result is smoother, softer, more glowing skin. The only downside with fruit enzymes is that they can be a bit acidic and might inflame sensitive skin.

RADIOFREQUENCY TREATMENT

Sofia Coppola has been a client and a friend of mine for almost a decade. We bonded immediately because we have daughters the same age, and we both love the world of beauty. When Sofia comes into the salon for a facial, we talk about our kids, as well as our favorite treatments, products, and all the ways we try to keep our skin looking great.

One summer, I got an email from Sofia saying she had experienced a treatment in France that had delivered incredible results in terms of skin tightening. (I love that when she travels, she tries new things and brings me back all the intel!) She was so excited about this treatment, called radiofrequency, that I knew I had to try it.

Honestly, radiofrequency treatment is as close to a noninvasive face-lift as I have ever seen. It's not a magic bullet—you need to do it as part of a series—but it really works, and it's one of the technologies I've been most excited about in the last few years. The term is certainly nothing new as far as science goes; we've understood for 150 years that energy can be measured in frequencies—meaning wavelengths per second—and that all frequencies lie on something we call the electromagnetic spectrum. Radio frequency is simply one of the categories on that spectrum, and it can exist as radio waves, Wi-Fi, television signals, and more.

Lest you get alarmed that you're going to microwave yourself or fry your brain if you apply radiofrequency to your face, let me put your fears to rest. In cosmetic treatments, the frequency we use is quite low. In fact, it's one *billion* times less powerful than an X-ray. But, like all energy, it produces heat, and that's where the amazing benefits of radiofrequency treatment start.

In my radiofrequency treatments, I use a small handheld wand with a rectangular head that distributes the energy directly onto the skin. If you've ever been pregnant, you'll probably remember that when you got an ultrasound, the tech slathered a cool, wet, colorless gel over your belly, then rubbed a wand across it. That's exactly what I do first: I dip the wand into sonogram gel, then move it in circular motions over your cheeks, eyes, nose, neck, and chin.

The warmth produced by radiofrequency literally heats the dermis and the subdermis, injuring the skin. When that happens, your body produces more collagen. In fact, radiofrequency causes you to produce 20 percent more collagen than you normally would! It also pushes the collagen fibers together, which helps thicken the skin. Immediately after a treatment, your skin will look plumper, more lifted, and firmer.

I also do radiofrequency treatments on my clients' butts, thighs, bellies, jawlines, and even their knees. When used with microneedling, it can help eliminate stretch marks anywhere on your body. Radiofrequency can also reduce the appearance of cellulite, because it helps thicken the thin skin, which hides the characteristic dimpled fat underneath. If you are concerned about a part of your body that sags or looks dimpled no matter how much you exercise, radiofrequency might be a good solution for you.

Radiofrequency treatment is not invasive, and it's not painful. Because there's heat, you may look red for about an hour post-treatment, but after that, you'll just be slightly pink. Some people may have spots afterward, but they're easy to cover up. Other than that, there are no negative side effects, and in fact, radiofrequency treatment can be positively life-changing. When we first got our radiofrequency machine at the salon, I invited some of my longtime clients in for a sneak-peek trial session. A few weeks later, a client who's close to sixty told me, "Joanna, thanks to radiofrequency, I don't feel invisible anymore!" It was one of those moments in my career that I will never forget.

The wonderful thing about this treatment is that it works whether you're twenty-five, eight-five, or somewhere in between. If your budget allows for it, I recommend having radiofrequency treatments once a week for eight weeks. If you're in your twenties, you might try doing it once every three months. At a minimum, radiofrequency treatment should be done once or twice a year.

• • •

WHAT ABOUT EXTRACTIONS?

In my decades as an aesthetician, one thing that's never changed is people's hatred of blackheads. Hands down, the first issue my clients mention when they come in for a facial are those gunky little dots that populate their faces like stars in the summer sky, making their pores look larger than they really are. My clients want extractions to get rid of blackheads, and they want them *now*.

Blackheads aren't a skin *problem*, per se—they are a natural by-product of your body's skin maintenance. You have hair follicles on every part of your skin except for your palms and the soles of your feet, and next to these follicles are sebaceous glands, which secrete sebum into the follicle. Now, here comes a big surprise: the pores on your face are actually *hair follicles*! And given their proximity to the sebaceous glands, it's no wonder that they become clogged up with sebum. Sure, foreign substances like pollution and makeup also clog your pores, but for the most part, the yucky stuff in blackheads is totally natural.

Even so, *everyone* wants them gone, and that's where the expertise of an aesthetician comes in. My first, very strong recommendation concerning extractions is this: do not do them at home! There's no substitute for a visit to a trained professional who has studied how to do extractions properly, hygienically, and in such a way that your pores will close after cleansing.

If you absolutely insist on the DIY route, here is my advice: Steam your face with a small steamer machine, or simply hop in a hot, steamy shower for a few minutes; the steam will loosen up the gunk in your pores. Then you can exfoliate, leaving your skin noticeably cleaner. If you like, follow up with a clay-based mask; simply blot your face dry with a clean towel and apply the mask to the areas where you have blackheads. (For most people, this is the nose, forehead, and chin.) Wait about ten minutes, then rinse your face with warm water. This process should gently clear blackheads, but if you try it and *still* have them, please don't reach for a set of tweezers or a double-edged blackhead extractor. These metal tools—which are made specifically for extractions and are available in almost every beauty aisle—can cause scarring, discoloration, and capillary damage, and can drive bacteria deeper into your flesh, leading to infection or inflammation. Instead, try holding a cotton swab in each hand and pressing them on either side of a blackhead. Don't squeeze too hard, as this can cause swelling—just press firmly directly alongside the blackhead until the dark, oily center pushes free of the pore.

Again, I hope you can schedule time for a facial if you feel you need extractions. Steaming, exfoliating, and applying a mask should make a noticeable difference and hold you over until you can see an aesthetician. Whatever you do, please resist the urge to use extraction tools, pick at your skin, or do anything else that might damage your beautiful face.

six

BETTER
SKIN NOW!

One of the first things I ask new clients when they come to see me is what their specific skincare needs are. Nine times out of ten, they tell me about a problem they're having. They might be troubled by dry, flaky patches; they could be shocked by the number of fine lines that have cropped up around their eyes; or maybe they've started having breakouts on skin that otherwise hadn't seen a pimple since puberty. Sometimes they know their routines have gone off the rails because they've been working too hard or just had a baby, but other times they're completely stumped because their skin has changed dramatically—

yet nothing about their lifestyle seems any different. I try to un-
cover the causes behind those mysteries, and then I work to fix
their skin woes by helping them reestablish good beauty habits and offering specific solutions. Those targeted tips are what I
want to share with you in this chapter. Think of this as a quick,
easy reference for troubleshooting the most common skincare
issues—the ones most people face at some time or another.

Of course, there is no one miracle cure as far as your skin is
concerned. You *must* take appropriate, long-term steps toward
fixing your diet, structuring a workable routine, and taking care
of yourself. But in a pinch, you can start with the troubleshooting
tips in this chapter.

targeted tips for . . .

ACNE

If you're troubled by acne and don't know where to turn, my first
recommendation is to take a close look at your diet. If you never
used to have breakouts but are now plagued by them, you might
have a sensitivity to casein, a protein found in milk. Try elimi-

glow from within

nating dairy and see if your skin clears up. Cut down on simple carbs (like bread) and sugar, which can lead to inflammation and excess sebum production, and add oily fish, green leafy vegetables, and a probiotic supplement to your diet.

In terms of clearing up existing acne, look for products that include salicylic acid, and avoid those with avocado oil, shea butter, or fatty acids. Try a using a clay mask a few times a week, especially one that contains zinc. You might also try a retinol, which can work miracles on acne-prone skin. Always use toner after cleansing to clear off excess oil and makeup, and dry your skin with disposable paper towels rather than a cloth towel.

If you can make an appointment at a spa, try a laser or LED light treatment. Not only do these cutting-edge therapies help clear up acne, but they're super relaxing and help cut down on the stress that can cause breakouts.

DARK CIRCLES

Because dark circles under your eyes can be the unfortunate by-products of heredity and aging, oftentimes there's no way to eliminate them completely. But you may be able to reduce their appearance with a few tweaks to your diet, lifestyle, and beauty routine.

Dark circles often form because your diet lacks enough vitamin K, potassium, and water. Try eating more leafy greens or a green juice with each meal, and increase your intake of water. Avoid caffeine and excess alcohol, which can constrict the blood vessels around your eyes, and cut out sugar and smoking. Lack of sleep is a huge cause of raccoon eyes, so be sure to rest as much as you can. Exercise can increase the blood flow to your face (and will also help you sleep).

Always, always wear eye cream, morning and night—especially an eye cream that contains peptides, almond oil, and vitamin E. If you're looking for a quick fix, put any kind of cold tea bags under your eyes, as the tannins in tea can lighten up dark spots. Cucumber slices will also hydrate your skin, as well as brighten it just a tad. You can also use avocado. Leave any of these ingredients on your closed eyes for about twenty minutes, then remove, rinse, and pat dry.

If you can make it to the spa, microneedling is terrific for dark circles, and your aesthetician can give you a lymphatic massage to help stimulate the flow of nutrients and blood to your eye area.

•   •   •

DRY, FLAKY PATCHES

You know what I'm talking about. They're those irritating little flakes of skin on your cheeks, forehead, the sides of your nose—anywhere, really—that sometimes appear out of nowhere. You might wonder, *How can I have one patch of flaky skin when the rest of my face seems fine?* Well, not all areas of skin react to stressors the same way, and dry patches may be the result of something bad happening on the inside of your body, or something that's negatively affecting it from the outside.

Regardless, there are plenty of things you can do about dry patches, beginning with making sure you're not dehydrated. Drink water consistently all day, and make sure you're not over-indulging in the alcohol department. Eat leafy greens, which are full of vitamins A and B; omega-3 fatty acids, which are found in oily fish; and biotin, which can be found in bananas, eggs, brown rice, and oatmeal (it can also be taken as a supplement). Flaky skin is sometimes just skin that's not receiving the nutrients it needs.

Intensely dry skin may be deprived of hyaluronic acid, so use products that contain it; it'll help lock in moisture in no time. You might also try shea butter, almond oil, or jojoba oil, whether in a serum or by themselves. Try a mask that contains avocado, or invest in a humidifier. Your skin may just be overly dry from the environment in which you're working or sleeping.

Finally, as our stress levels increase, so does cortisol in our systems, and this reduces the level of hyaluronic acid in the body. Managing the stress in your life will help clear up your skin.

DULLNESS

A buildup of dead skin cells coupled with slow cell turnover can leave your skin looking tired and dull. To combat this, make sure you're drinking enough water; your skin could be dehydrated. Cut back on alcohol and excess caffeine, and avoid processed sugars, which cause collagen breakdown and slow cell turnover.

Be sure that you're cleansing in two steps: first removing makeup and environmental debris, and then using a mild cleanser. A toner with a mild exfoliant like papaya enzyme or lactic acid may complete this process, leading to a smooth, clear palette. Most important, exfoliate at least two times a week; this will sweep away the dead cells that are making your skin look dull. Follow with a clay mask or one that contains glycolic acid or galactoarabinan.

glow from within

When you moisturize, look for products that contain hyaluronic acid, which will help your skin retain moisture (giving you a dewy glow), as well as protect you against free radical damage from environmental stressors. If you have a little extra to spend, seek out products with epidermal growth factors (EGFs), or schedule a facial with an oxygen treatment.

ECZEMA

Eczema is caused by inflammation, so the first thing you need to do is look at your diet and determine if anything you're eating might be triggering inflammation in your body. Are you relying on a lot of processed foods or eating more gluten or sugar than usual? Limiting these inflammatory foods can help keep the red, scaly, itchy patches characteristic of eczema at bay. Add probiotics to your diet as well; I've seen remarkable results, in both the short and long terms, when people suffering from this super-irritating condition up their intake of yogurt, fermented foods, or probiotic supplements. Finally, be sure the foods you're eating contain enough zinc, which is found in animal proteins, almonds, asparagus, and spinach. If you're worried you aren't getting enough zinc, try a supplement.

Lighter facial oils, including marula and flaxseed oils, are great for hydration and for clearing up eczema. Be sure to use them in combination with your regular moisturizer for maximum effect.

OILINESS

One of the easiest ways to determine if your skin classifies as oily is to look at your face about an hour after you wash it. Is it shiny? Then you have oily skin! But contrary to popular belief, excessively oily skin doesn't need to be dried out or stripped of oil—it requires ingredients and products that are calming. It may also need moisturizer, so try something with glycolic acid or jojoba oil, which will help maintain your skin's natural balance of sebum.

While many people only wash their skin at night, that's a no-no for people with oily complexions. Try an oil-based cleanser that contains hazelnut, castor, grape seed, or jojoba oil (all of which break up oils and impurities), or opt for cleansers with glycolic or salicylic acid in them. Dry your face with a paper towel rather than a cloth towel, and follow with toner, which is a must for removing that final layer of oil and debris. Do *not* overexfoliate, a common mistake many people with oily skin make. Exfoliate just once or twice a week with a salicylic acid–based scrub, and indulge yourself with a clay-based mask, especially one that contains zinc, jojoba oil, or kaolin clay.

Excess sebum production may be the result of stress or inflammation, so engage in good self-care techniques, and cut back on foods that cause inflammation.

PSORIASIS

The itchy, scaly, red-and-white patches of skin caused by psoriasis can be among the most frustrating skin issues in the world—but they don't have to be the *end* of the world. Psoriasis, an auto-immune disorder that causes a massive buildup of cells directly on the skin's surface, can in some cases be successfully alleviated through a combination of diet, good products, and lifestyle adjustments. The omega-3 fatty acids in oily fish, walnuts, leafy greens, and pumpkin can slow your immune system's overactive response, and taking probiotics regularly can further halt it. Oftentimes, psoriasis sufferers know the triggers that will cause an outbreak—typically overindulging in fatty and sugary foods or alcohol, stress, lack of sleep, sunburn, or sickness—so staying healthy, practicing good self-care, and wearing sunscreen will help prevent outbreaks.

If you do have an outbreak, good moisturizers—especially those containing hyaluronic acid, which will help you retain moisture—can lessen its severity. Soothing ingredients such as avocado and oatmeal can help as well. If all else fails and you have recurring outbreaks, seek help from an aesthetician or dermatologist. Psoriasis can be a lifelong condition, but it is much more manageable if you've got a good team on your side.

PUFFINESS

You're bloated all over your body, and the area around your eyes looks twice its normal size. What's going on here? You've got a major case of puffiness, and I can promise you it's got something to do with your diet. General bloat in the body or the face can be brought on by a diet too high in sodium, which causes you to retain water. You may be the kind of person who doesn't even own a saltshaker, much less crave salty foods, but sodium is hidden in all kinds of foods, including snack foods, canned goods, soups, sauces, and condiments. Restaurant food is also typically high in sodium, so if you're going out to eat or ordering takeout frequently, you're probably eating a lot of salt. If you don't drink enough water to flush it out, your body will retain water, and you'll look puffy.

One of the best ways to get rid of the bloat is to exercise. Moving your body gets your blood flowing, allowing much-needed nutrients and water to circulate. Eating something green at every meal will get your lymphatic system pumping, which will flush out the impurities that keep you puffy. Try lymphatic massage if you're experiencing puffiness on your face, and if it's all over your body, dry brush every day. Again, this will get your lymphatic and circulatory systems moving.

Good-quality products can help diminish puffiness as well. Dab a high-quality eye cream around your eyes morning and night, and use a moisturizer that helps maintain a good overall moisture balance, especially one that contains hyaluronic acid.

ROSACEA

The red, bumpy, or spidery areas you see on your upper cheeks might make you look like you're either embarrassed or overexerted, but the truth is that they're usually the result of a common skin condition called rosacea. Rosacea is caused by inflammation, so chances are, you're likely experiencing a sensitivity to dairy, sugar, or grain, or inflammation from consuming alcohol or sugar. Try cutting back on any or all of those and see if the rosacea subsides.

If it doesn't, eating probiotic foods or taking a probiotic supplement can go a long way. Drinking coffee might help to decrease the redness because coffee constricts the blood vessels. Try applying products containing hyaluronic acid, aloe, lavender, or rose hip oil, which will soothe the skin and help it maintain its overall balance. If you have time and money to go to the spa, LED light therapy can greatly help diminish rosacea, too.

This terrific little at-home remedy for rosacea is easy to make and will help improve your symptoms right away.

Constriction Prescription for Reducing Redness

2 cups distilled water
1 cup lavender flowers
1 ounce fresh peppermint leaves
4 teaspoons green tea
2 teaspoons fresh or pure aloe vera gel

In a small saucepan, bring the water to a boil. Remove from the heat and add the lavender, peppermint, and tea.

glow from within

Let steep for 15 minutes, then strain the mixture through a fine-mesh strainer into a bowl, discarding the solids, and let it cool completely. Stir in the aloe vera gel and pour into a spray bottle (preferably made of glass). Mist it on your face a few times a day. I do not recommend storing food masks in the refrigerator; instead, make them from scratch each time you plan to use them.

For an on-the-go version: Place 1 organic peppermint tea bag and 1 chamomile teabag in a cup of warm water and let steep until the water has cooled. Add the aloe vera gel, stir, and pour into a spray bottle.

SENSITIVE SKIN

"Sensitive skin" is really a blanket term for any kind of irritation your skin experiences from an external or internal force, and it encompasses everything from redness to bumpiness to a full-on pimply breakout. Preventing sensitive skin is all about avoiding the products and foods that trigger your skin problems—and using products and foods that won't.

What are these foods and ingredients that might lead to issues? They include all the usual suspects, like sugar, alcohol, processed foods, dairy, and highly processed grains, all of which may cause an allergic response in the body. Try cutting back or eliminating some of them and see if your sensitivities clear up. Because fragrances, parabens, sulfates, dyes, chemical sunscreens, physical exfoliants (i.e., scrubs), and retinol are all common irritants, you might want to avoid some or all of these as well.

People with sensitive skin need calming, soothing ingredients from plant-based products. Cleansing balms that contain sweet almond oil, cocoa butter, shea butter, glycerin, ceramides, or hyaluronic acid are often soothing, and cleansers with oleic, palmitic, or linoleic fatty acids calm the skin. Try a soothing cream mask with avocado, shea butter, chamomile, arnica, aloe, or sulfur, and moisturize with avocado, coconut, or jojoba oil. Most of all, just monitor your skin—if you notice that using a specific product (which could be any household item from laundry detergent to dish soap) seems to be connected with a skin issue, cut it out.

Model Tess Holliday, one of my clients, often has breakouts because of her sensitive skin. Tess is a bombshell even when she's off duty. What's even more interesting is that she is equal parts intelligent, sweet, and thoughtful, and from the beginning of an appointment to the end, we never stop talking, laughing, and analyzing everything.

When I first met her, she was struggling to find products that worked for her. Her beauty routine was great in theory, but her skin wasn't responding to it. While other people had suggested that her skin troubles were lifestyle related (working and traveling all the time, not getting enough sleep, eating on the go, etc.), as a facialist, it's my job to suggest a good routine that is tailored to my client's lifestyle, not suggest they quit their job! I suspected that her sensitivities had a lot to do with all the makeup she wore, and we needed a way to protect her skin and help it recover. My solution was for Tess to use a healing, anti-inflammatory vitamin C oil, followed by a soothing sheet mask before she goes into hair and makeup. Her skin has vastly improved on this new routine. Today, I am proud every time Tess posts a makeup-free selfie!

UNEVEN SKIN TONE

Uneven skin tone, hyperpigmentation, brown spots, or melasma—brownish-gray patches found on the face, arms, or neck—are some of the hallmarks of the aging process. Luckily, there are effective treatments for all of them—but first you have to understand how and why these conditions develop.

As we age and the level of hyaluronic acid in our skin decreases, our cells aren't able to retain water the way they did before. This leads to slower cell turnover and patchy, dull skin.

Using a moisturizer with hyaluronic acid and exfoliating two or three times a week will encourage cell turnover and pave the way for fresher, clearer skin with a more consistent tone.

Uneven tone may also be the result of high estrogen levels, which are frequently caused by hormonal contraceptives or estrogen replacement treatments. If you're taking estrogen or using a hormone-based contraceptive and have noticed that your skin looks different, talk to your gynecologist; maybe estrogen isn't for you, or maybe you've been prescribed too much or it.

The most common cause of brown spots, melasma, and hyperpigmentation is sun damage. While it's impossible to completely reverse the harm caused by the sun, laser and LED light treatments can help tremendously. Talk to an aesthetician and see if these treatments are right for you.

I've known actress Haley Bennett, another client of mine, for a very long time. Haley has beautiful, milky skin with a sprinkling of freckles on her nose. But like many fair or freckled people—including myself—she sometimes struggles with melasma. Like me, Haley will get a Clear + Brilliant laser treatment once a year to stay on top of any sun damage. In combination with wearing sunscreen and a hat, and getting regular facials and LED light therapy, she can prevent uneven skin tone and maintain her movie star glow.

WRINKLES AND FINE LINES

I could write an entire book on how to reduce wrinkles (and maybe someday I will!). The reality is that fine lines are an inevitable result of the aging process. But while you can't erase them or prevent them from developing, there are many noninvasive techniques you can employ to minimize their appearance and keep them at bay for as long as possible.

Start by looking at your diet. Are you drinking enough water? Dehydrated skin will purse up and wrinkle, so you *must* stay well hydrated at all times. Make sure you're eating plenty of healthy sources of omega-3, omega-6, and omega-9 fatty acids, which help your body retain moisture, fight inflammation, and improve cell function and structure (for a descrition of some of these foods, turn to page 28). A sufficient supply of zinc can help build up collagen in your skin, which gives you a full, radiant-rather-than-wrinkly look, while selenium and vitamin E, which are found in many types of fish, can also help fight the effects of aging. Avoid excess alcohol and caffeine, which can dehydrate your skin, leading to the formation of wrinkles.

My number one wrinkle-fighting tip, however, is to wear sunscreen. Hands down, sun damage is the primary cause of wrinkles and fine lines, and if you start wearing adequate sun protection when you're young, you'll look great as you age. Parents: Always put sunscreen on your kids! It will instill good habits in them for the rest of their lives.

If you do have pesky wrinkles or fine lines, products containing lactic acid, glycolic acid, or antioxidants like vitamins C and E (which helps build up collagen) will visibly reduce them. I love using a vitamin C face wash, then following it with a moisturizer containing hyaluronic acid. Exfoliate at least two or three times a week, which will clear away your dead skin cells, make way for new skin cells that are able to retain moisture, and instantly give you clearer, plumper skin. Finally, if you don't have overly sensitive skin, retinol can work wonders.

If you can make it to the spa, try an LED light therapy facial, microneedling, or microdermabrasion. Together or separately, these techniques will stop wrinkles in their tracks and help prevent the formation of new ones.

glow from within

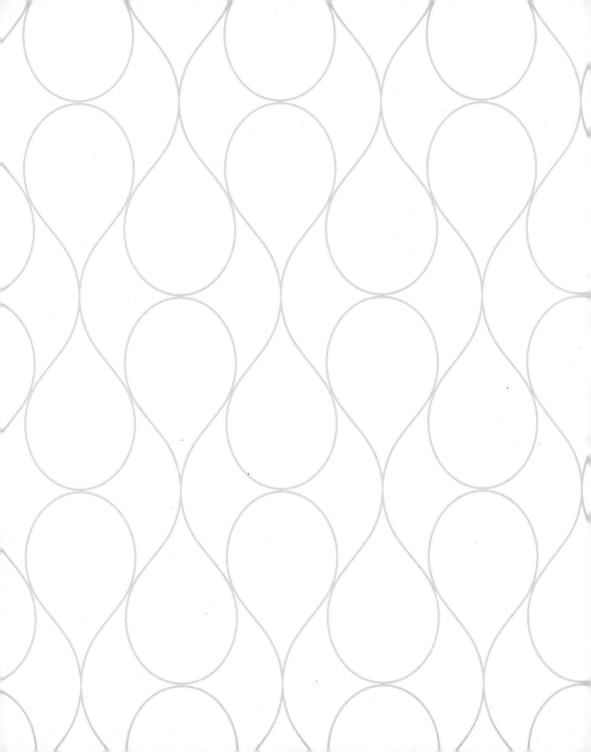

seven

TIME-
TARGETED
ROUTINES
FOR
FLAWLESS
SKIN

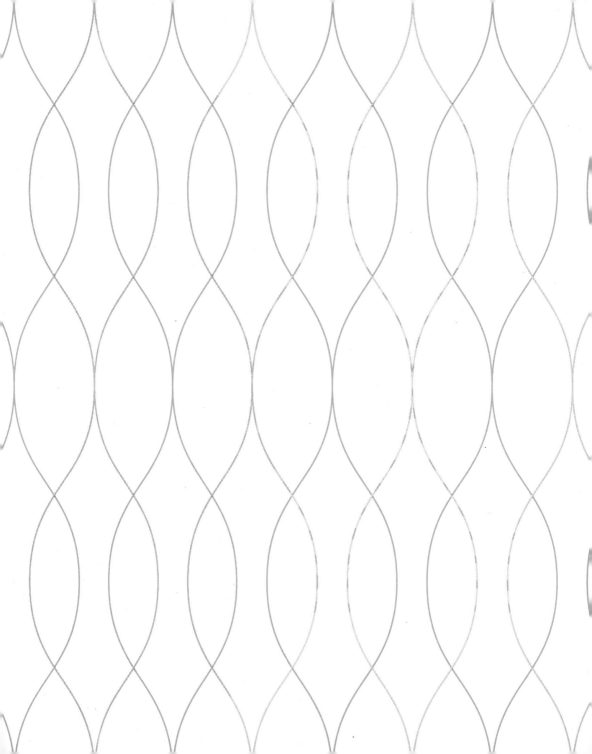

At my salons, we see a lot of clients who are prepping for a big event: a wedding, a reunion, a dream vacation, or some other special moment for which they desperately want to look their best. It's my job to listen to their goals and figure out how I can help achieve them in the quickest, easiest way possible. Getting first-date or red-carpet ready on schedule is a priority for almost everyone at some point in their lives, so this section will show you how to implement a time-sensitive routine, whether you have six months or one day.

The clock is ticking, so get ready! It's time to look gorgeous.

six months to glowing skin

Six months is a perfect amount of time to completely restructure your habits to create the best version of you. What I'm about to present is a workable routine you can follow no matter your skin type—but you *must* do it every day, no matter how tired you are!

The first thing you need to address is your nightly routine. Double cleansing nightly with micellar water and a foaming face wash, or using a cleansing balm for makeup removal followed by a foaming face wash, is important. I would also start using a retinol at night twice a week at first, then, if your skin reacts well, every other day, then a week or so later, daily. Finish your routine with some type of hydrating serum/cream on top of the retinol for maximum repair and resurfacing.

In the morning, start using a hyaluronic serum that contains greens, like oat grass juice or chlorophyll, for light hydration and oxygenation, followed by a moisturizer and sunscreen with an SPF of 30. Twice a week, exfoliate and apply a sheet mask. Sheet masks that have hyaluronic acid, EGFs, peptides, antioxidants, and soothing ingredients like chamomile are helpful to your routine no matter your skin type.

Don't forget to give yourself a lymphatic massage as often as

glow from within

you can, even during hormonal fluctuations. It will go a long way to keeping your skin clear and glowing throughout the month. If possible, also try to get a facial once a month to clean out your pores. A microcurrent facial with some extractions and a hydrating balancing mask are great steps for anyone to take. The results of the microcurrent therapy are cumulative, so getting a treatment regularly for six months before a big day will lead to steady—yet dramatic—results. If you want a more serious investment, spend six months doing a series of radiofrequency facials, which I consider the most dramatic noninvasive treatment in the beauty industry.

Take a long, hard look at your diet. If you break out, are there triggers? Do you tend to eat poorly if alcohol is involved? Quitting drinking for a period of time is not only healthy—it may give you the strength you need to make real changes in how you treat yourself. Eating greens with every meal is a must. Greens contain essential minerals and vitamins for your skin and lymphatic system. If you hate eating veggies, then at least drink a shot of chlorophyll, which is equivalent to three servings of greens. Buying liquid chlorophyll is an easy way to get an extra dose of greens in your body even before you start your day. It will energize your cells, oxygenate, mineralize, activate your lymphatic system, de-puff you, and give you a healthy glow.

When I am treating an actress during awards season, we start working together for the film premiere, then the press tour, and finally for all the award shows. These women are flying everywhere, not sleeping well, and often not eating well, either. This kind of high-stress, nonstop activity isn't unique to famous people, though. Just about every woman I know lives some version of this life, and when we start to feel run-down physically and energetically, our confidence plummets. Instead of focusing on the negative or getting mired in self-criticism, I encourage all my clients to make small, healthy changes that get them back to a better place, and try their best to focus their energy on positive things in the meantime. Mental stress is only going to make everything—including your skin—worse.

Finally, when you're preparing for a big day, I encourage you to look at your schedule and see where you can fit in time for relaxation. Can you stop watching TV before bed and read a book to give yourself a break from electronics? You will fall asleep faster and have more restful beauty sleep. Can you put away your phone ten minutes earlier and spend that time meditating or listening to music? I paint and draw in the evenings, and I find that both activities really relax me. I don't check email after a certain hour. I spend time with my family. I used to have restless nights filled with tension; now I can't keep my eyes open. Find what makes you happy—your face will show it.

one month to glowing skin

One month till a huge event in your life is crunch time! But don't worry—it's not too late to completely transform your skin.

Your first step is twice-a-week exfoliation and hydration at home. Exfoliation is the key to glowing, clean skin, and I have told many people that a great exfoliator is a facial in a jar. Using one with both a scrub component and an acid/enzyme component makes it easy to use on all skin types. Scrub in areas where you feel you have a buildup of blackheads or clogged pores and then leave a thin layer on all over. Don't forget your neck and décolletage! After all, that's what usually shows when you are wearing a killer dress. Follow each exfoliation with a sheet mask, because it's important to nourish and hydrate after resurfacing the skin.

I would not start a retinol serum this close to your big day. But don't feel like you're missing out. You can simply use a vitamin

C serum at night for maximum repair and healing while you sleep. Vitamin C is the most healing ingredient we have at our disposal, and it's agreeable with any skin type. I would invest in a good formula, because this is your one-month-away secret weapon. You will be glowing for miles!

Your daytime routine will be similar to the one I outlined in the six-month program: serum, moisture, and sunscreen. The other thing I want to stress to you is WEAR A HAT! Not only can sun damage the skin and age us prematurely, but it will also completely destroy all the good you've done with your careful exfoliation and skin nourishing. Invest in a chic hat, and wear it every time you leave the house.

For your diet, I would strongly suggest you consider giving up gluten, dairy, and sugar for the month. None of these do anything positive for you or your skin. This goes for alcohol, too. All of my stressed-out brides give up alcohol a month before their big day. Who needs the bloat? It's not worth it! Besides, nothing feels better than knowing you've loved yourself and tried your hardest to feel your best for whatever event you were prepping for. Every time you look back at your photos, you'll smile, knowing that you took care of yourself.

I would also consider giving yourself a lymphatic massage daily, which will ensure a de-puffed, relaxed, oxygenated, and glowing face. Doing it before bed helps you have a less puffy visage when you wake up, too. Don't forget your eye area; it should get some de-puffing stimulation as well.

Finally, don't forget about the skin that's not on your face. Your skin is an organ, after all. I would start by dry brushing daily in the morning before jumping in the shower—you will see a difference in two weeks' time. Finish with a nice body cream containing antioxidants, cocoa butter, shea butter, peptides, and hyaluronic acid. These ingredients are great for keeping the skin supple, smooth, and glowing all over.

one week to glowing skin

When you have only a week to prepare your skin, I would not recommend using any new products or getting a facial anywhere you've never gotten one before. The stakes are too high, and too much can go wrong. But there are plenty of other things you can do to boost your glow in just a few days.

First, I would start drinking chlorophyll every morning to improve digestion, reduce inflammation, and introduce vitamins and minerals to the body. If you haven't already, lay off alcohol, breads, pastas, sugars, and dairy, too. It's just one week, and it might save you from getting a last-minute breakout or uneven skin. Makeup will also go on easier, and you won't feel puffy.

If your skin is tired or dull, exfoliate with your regular exfoliating product at least twice this week. This final week is *not* the time to experiment with a whole new routine, but exfoliation will ensure your products penetrate better and leave the skin resurfaced and more even.

I would also use a sheet mask (one you have used before without issue) the night before and on the morning of your big day. Sheet masks are prescriptive, so use a soothing one the night before and a hydrating EGF/peptide mask the morning of the event. They'll make a big difference.

The night before, you should absolutely use a body scrub to make the skin on your body smoother and more radiant. If you don't have a scrub on hand, you can make this simple one to use on both your face and your body. It smells like heaven and makes the skin feel smoother without irritating it.

* * *

Skin Smoother/Resurfacing Mask

1 cup brown sugar
¼ cup honey
¼ cup olive oil

If your skin is feeling super dry anytime during the week, you can also make a quick hydrating mask: mash an avocado with 1 cup plain yogurt, apply the mixture to your skin, and leave it on for fifteen minutes, then rinse.

tips for tonight

You've got a hot date in T-minus one day. What should you do *right now*?

First things first: Keep up your regular nighttime routine, starting with a thorough cleansing to remove the day's makeup and pollution. Sleep in a mask (if you don't have a full night to prepare, just apply a mask now and keep it on for as long as possible). If your skin is dry, use a nighttime hydrating mask. As you apply your mask, do a face massage. From the neck upward, from inside to outside, move your fingers in small circles, which will encourage lymphatic drainage and stimulate circulation. If you're broken out, dot a clay mask onto your blemishes and leave it on as a spot treatment; it will help heal the breakout overnight.

Get seven to eight hours of sleep! It's what your body needs. If you have trouble falling asleep, make yourself a nice cup of chamomile tea or a calcium/magnesium drink, or take a low dose of melatonin that will help knock you out. I also find that wearing a sleep mask over my eyes keeps me asleep and in a much deeper, more restful sleep zone.

When you're showering the day before or the day of, using a nice body scrub exfoliates your skin and brings out its glow. Gently scrub your entire body, including your face, for a solid ten minutes while you're in the shower. This will remove surface dirt, clean out your pores, and even your skin tone, just like a mini facial! Next, apply a great hydrating mask if you have normal or dry skin, or a clay mask if you are struggling with breakouts.

As you are applying your skincare products the day of, do another face massage. Again, this will reduce puffiness and make your skin look brighter and better, even under makeup.

Now go out and enjoy!

afterword

COSMETIC PROCEDURES— SHOULD YOU OR SHOULDN'T YOU?

One of the questions my clients ask me most often is "Should I get cosmetic surgery?" Unfortunately, there's no easy, straightforward answer for this. First of all, cosmetic surgery encompasses a range of treatments—from injectables like Botox to fillers like Juvéderm and Restylane to inpatient surgeries like face-lifts—so I never approach the subject as if there's a one-size-fits-all answer. If my client is seventy-five years old and desperately unhappy about her sagging jawline, and I'm certain that no amount of LED light therapy is going to make a noticeable difference, I'll be honest that a little nip and tuck might be right for her. However, if a forty-year-old woman with a few fine lines on her forehead complains that nothing but Botox will help her get rid of them, I'll tell her she's wrong. She's young, and with a little patience, effort, and help from me, she can minimize the appearance of her wrinkles without resorting to Botox. It's true! Even though the use of minimally invasive cosmetic treatments has grown a whopping 200 percent since 2000 and the taboo around them is almost entirely gone, I don't believe that most women need these kinds of interventions to achieve the results they want. A consistent skincare routine, regular facials, a great diet, and good self-care will produce results that are just as satisfying.

However, we live in a world obsessed with instant gratification—where you can buy a car and have it delivered to your door, or find a date just by swiping right on your phone—so many people think that a quick fix is the only fix. It's not; cosmetic surgery can alter the way you look in ways you may not anticipate or want. Sure, injectables will deliver a wrinkle-free forehead in only a few days, but they may also give you a frozen, deer-in-the-headlights look. Getting a fast, easy solution also tends to make women go overboard, thinking that physical perfection is the only answer for them. They might look at a star's puffy pout on Instagram and run to their dermatologist for some instant plumping, but larger lips may not actually suit their face. Worst of all, cosmetic surgery can have terrible side effects, like bleeding, scarring, bruising, numbness, pain, and decreased mobility. This doesn't happen in an aesthetician's salon. I promise you, no one has ever left me with a swollen, bleeding face! Instead, I work tirelessly to give my clients the tools to become, over time, the best, most natural versions of themselves.

If you do consider cosmetic surgery, find a surgeon or dermatologist who isn't afraid to offer you other alternatives. No doctor should be eager to cut into your face just because you think that's what you want. In addition, any good cosmetic dermatologist or plastic surgeon should ask you about the state of your mental health to make sure you're in the right frame of mind to make such a big decision.

Surgery is a last resort, and I hope this book has shown you the many ways you can achieve a healthy, glow-from-within look without it. You are gorgeous inside and out, and I sincerely hope I've opened up the world of safe, natural skincare to you so that you can make the best decisions for yourself. When it comes to beauty, knowledge is power—and the power is in your hands.

ACKNOWLEDGMENTS

In many ways, this book is a dream come true for me. As with everything I have done, I have many people to thank.

To my husband, Cesar: thank you for always believing in me and always pushing me to be the best version of myself. You are a partner in everything I have accomplished in life. You are the best CEO, the best husband, and the best father.

To my children, Odin and Ruby: everything I do in life is for you. You guys are and continue to be my true inspiration. I love you both so much.

To Tara Lowenberg, my sister, friend, and the world's best publicist: thank you for always having my back in everything I do. And to Tara Yamaoka, my PR team leader: thank you for always executing the best plans with the best smile and never letting anything ruffle your feathers.

To Christina Han, my first and best beauty industry friend: Your friendship and endless support mean so much to me.

To Dr. Frank Lipman: thank you for your friendship and for always being there whenever I need you.

To Melissa Ouelette, Krista Lavrusik, and my dearest departed Lena Vitolo: I cannot put into words how much you mean to me. Without you I would not have grown into who I am today. Your hard work resonates throughout the hallways of our salon. I wouldn't be here without you, and I am so blessed to know that I still have you guys by my side in everything to come.

To Kimberly Gutzmore, for being my ride or die across the world and back again.

To my incomparable staff, whose trust, hard work, intelligence, and excellence always make me proud.

To Aviva B, Robin K, Lois Z, Vivian K, Page H, Susan C, and Sammie B, who supported me and believed in me when no one else did.

To Theresa Coffino, for your endless support of all my new creations.

To my entire team at HarperWave: Julie Will, you were my dream editor, and I couldn't imagine doing this project with anyone else. To Haley Swanson, Bonni Leon-Berman, Yelena Nesbit, Nikki Baldauf, Penny Makras, and Caroline Johnson: you all have the hearts of artists, and for that I am forever grateful.

Sarah Durand, the woman who helped turn my vision into reality: Thank you for making the writing of this book come true. Your experience, talent, and wisdom are unmatched, and I can't thank you enough for being a part of this with me.

To my agent, Stephanie Tade: Thank you for your endless positivity and guidance throughout the entire journey.

Thank you to all my friends and family for being my biggest cheerleaders.

And finally, to my grandmother: Thank you for always letting me play with all your beauty products, for teaching me my first lessons in skincare, and being the ultimate beauty icon for me. I owe my passion for the industry to you.

appendix
RECIPES

juices

Not a day goes by when I don't drink a green juice with at least one of my meals. Green juice provides you with essential vitamins and minerals. It also instantly hydrates the skin while encouraging lymphatic drainage. The three recipes that follow are variations on one another, offering similar benefits but containing different ingredients. You will need a juicer to make these, but if you don't have one, just request these blends at your local juice bar!

Mrs. Clean

This crisp, refreshing juice (with a slight zing!) will help flush your lymph.

    10 celery stalks
    1 small bunch parsley
    1/3 medium cucumber
    1/4 medium apple
    Juice of 1 lemon
    Grated fresh ginger

Miracle Clean

This juice will transform you from under the weather to strong and vibrant. Cilantro is a powerful antioxidant that also acts as a diuretic. It reduces puffiness associated with your monthly cycle, detoxes heavy metals, lowers blood sugar levels, and makes the urinary tract healthier.

    2 carrots
    1 medium apple

2 bunches cilantro

1 small bunch parsley

Juice of 1 lemon

1 teaspoon grated fresh ginger

Perfectly Clean

Think of this as a multivitamin in a glass, or your extra salad of the day to keep the doctor away. This well-balanced juice provides antioxidants, beta carotene, fiber, vitamin A, and more.

4 celery stalks

2 carrots

2 medium beets

1/3 medium cucumber

1 small bunch parsley

2 handfuls of spinach

Handful of kale

Juice of 1 lemon

1 teaspoon grated fresh ginger

masks

There's really nothing more soothing for your face than a mask. Masks moisturize, de-puff, promote elasticity, and relieve skin sensitivities. The fifteen to twenty minutes you spend wearing a mask is also time you're forced to drop all chores and errands and just sit back and relax. If you don't have masks at home, you can easily make them with the following simple recipes. Just combine the ingredients in a small bowl and mix to form a paste. For one minute, rub the paste onto your skin using the tips of your fingers in upward strokes, then leave it on for ten to fifteen minutes. Rinse with tepid water. Food ingredients can spoil, so don't store what you have left over or make a mask a day in advance. Instead, mix up a fresh mask every time you plan to use one.

Antioxidant/Antiaging Mask

This light, oily mask hydrates, tightens pores, and reduces inflammation, making your skin noticeably brighter. The almond meal exfoliates, smoothing out wrinkles to help turn back the clock.

2 tablespoons grape seed oil
5 teaspoons almond meal
1 teaspoon warmed honey
2 drops rose oil

Hydrating Mask

The name says it all! This creamy mask soothes, moisturizes, and feels like butter on your skin.

½ cup plain yogurt
½ avocado
¼ cup honey

Cooling Mask

Rich in aloe vera, this soothing mask is perfect if you've spent too long in the sun. The oat or wheat grass detoxes, stimulates the lymphatic system, and gives your tired skin the nutrients it needs.

    ¼ cup plain yogurt
    3 tablespoons fresh or pure aloe vera gel
    2 tablespoons oat grass juice or wheat grass juice

Clear Skin Mask

If you're bothered by persistent breakouts or dull, oily skin, this soothing mask will help brighten, clear, and reduce surface bacteria.

    1 cup plain yogurt
    ½ cup strawberries, mashed
    ½ cup almond meal
    Raw apple cider vinegar

appendix: recipes

In a small bowl, stir together the yogurt, strawberries, and almond meal.

Dip a cotton ball in vinegar and rub it over the area that is breaking out. Immediately apply the mask, using upward strokes, and leave it on for 10 to 15 minutes, then rinse.

Hydrating Spice Mask

Nourishing, anti-inflammatory, and rich in nutrients that stimulate the lymphatic system, this mask smells absolutely divine! It's ideal if you're looking for an invigorating, hydrating glow.

1/2 avocado
1 tablespoon manuka honey
2 teaspoons coconut oil
1/2 teaspoon fresh fennel, chopped

Brightening Antioxidant Mask

As deliciously smooth and satisfying as a cup of hot cocoa, this hydrating mask evens out your pigment and reduces inflammation and redness. Perfect for anyone with rosacea or dull, sensitive skin.

3 tablespoons honey
1 teaspoon unsweetened cocoa powder
1 teaspoon ground nutmeg
1 teaspoon ground cinnamon

Matcha Glow Mask

Is your skin looking dull and tired, with a noticeable lack of suppleness? This light mask strengthens your capillary walls and increases circulation, giving your skin a smooth, pillowy softness.

1½ teaspoons water
1 tablespoon matcha powder
1½ teaspoons honey
1 tablespoon olive oil

Add water and matcha powder first, stir, then add other ingredients and combine.

Cocoa and Champagne Mask

If you suffer from frequent breakouts, this soothing, hydrating mask will tone your skin and reduce inflammation, giving you a brighter, younger appearance.

½ cup plain yogurt
¼ cup champagne
1 tablespoon unsweetened cocoa powder
1 tablespoon honey

Cranberry Mask

If you've been outside, battling the elements, your skin may look as worn out as you are. This wrinkle-fighting mask boosts collagen production, diminishes the appearance of wrinkles, and prevents free radical damage.

½ cup pureed cranberries
3 tablespoons plain yogurt
1 tablespoon coconut oil
1 tablespoon honey

Brightening Mask

Does your skin need instant glow? This silky mask will give you bright, pliable, hydrated skin in no time.

  1 tablespoon green tea, made fresh from
      loose leaves or a tea bag
  2 teaspoons honey
  2 teaspoons plain yogurt
  1 teaspoon coconut oil

Milk and Honey Glow Mask

This rich, creamy mask is as soothing as they come. Perfect for dull, overtaxed skin, it softens and calms redness, giving you a much-needed boost.

  ½ teaspoon brown sugar
  ½ cup cooked oatmeal
  ¼ cup honey
  ¼ cup milk

Pumpkin Mask

Summer is over, so it's time to repair your sun-damaged skin. Bring on the pumpkin! This mask provides restorative nutrients as it soothes and hydrates.

  2 teaspoons pure pumpkin puree
  1 teaspoon plain yogurt
  ½ teaspoon honey

Pineapple Enzyme Mask

If you have dull, sensitive skin, this mask—rich in fruit enzymes—will exfoliate, resurface, and stimulate your lymphatic system, restoring your glow.

  ¼ cup pineapple, mashed
  2 tablespoons almond meal
  1 teaspoon coconut milk

Chia Seed Mask

This is a great all-around mask that can be used anytime to calm, soothe, and provide essential fatty acids to the skin.

2 tablespoons coconut oil
1 tablespoon ground chia seeds
1 teaspoon matcha powder

Bee Pollen Superfood Mask

Look forever young with this mask! Bee pollen contains nucleic acid, which prevents premature aging and stimulates cell renewal.

1 tablespoon avocado, mashed
1 teaspoon bee pollen
1 teaspoon coconut oil, melted
1 teaspoon honey

Citrus and Oatmeal Mask

This thick, creamy mask is a delicious, vitamin-boosting breakfast for your face. Apply in the morning to soothe, calm, exfoliate, and get your face ready for the day.

    2 tablespoons plain cottage cheese
    2 tablespoons cooked oatmeal
    ¼ orange, peeled, seeded, and mashed

Creamy Hydrating Mask

This simple mask hydrates and repairs dry skin with vitamin A and potassium. It's a perfect, quick way to give yourself a nutrient-rich moisturizing boost.

    ½ banana, mashed
    2 tablespoons plain cottage cheese
    1 teaspoon honey

Antiaging Mask

If you've looked in the mirror and fretted over your fine lines and wrinkles, mix up this mask and apply it regularly. It lightly exfoliates while reducing inflammation and fighting sun damage.

> 2 tablespoons honey
> 1 tablespoon brown sugar
> 1½ teaspoons cumin seed oil
> 1 teaspoon olive oil

Anti-Inflammatory Mask

If you've partied too hard, slept too little, or worked too much, this mask is for you. The ginger reduces puffiness and increases collagen, while the almond meal exfoliates and stimulates your lymphatic system.

> ¼ cup coconut oil
> 1 tablespoon grated fresh ginger
> 1 tablespoon almond meal

appendix: recipes

GLOSSARY
OF
SKIN TERMS

Antioxidants: Molecules that prevent cellular damage by free radicals. They may be produced within the body or derived from the food you eat.

Collagen: The most abundant protein in the human body, making up 25 to 35 percent of the body's total proteins. It forms the connective tissue for our skin, muscles, tendons, ligaments, and more.

Dermis: The thickest layer of the skin, which lies under the epidermis and above the subcutaneous fat layer. Containing blood vessels, oil and sweat glands, nerves, lymphatic vessels, and hair follicles, it provides structure and stability to the skin.

Eczema: A skin condition caused by inflammation and characterized by red, itchy, dry patches.

Elastin: The elastic protein found especially within the connective tissue of the dermis that allows your skin to stretch and bounce back.

Epidermis: The top layer of the skin, which provides protection against water loss, bacteria, viruses, the rays of the sun, and environmental pollutants.

Free radicals: Highly unstable molecules that have lost electrons; they attack and damage cells within your body. Formed when your body comes into contact with environmental stressors or germs, or when your diet is poor.

Keratin: A fibrous structural protein found in the surface cells of your hair, skin, nails, internal organs, and glands. It provides structure and resilience, and helps prevent cell damage.

Keratinocytes: The most common type of skin cells, they produce keratin.

Lymphatic system: Part of the vascular and immune systems, it's the network of tissues, organs, glands, and vessels that clears your body of toxins, drains tissues, and maintains your body's fluid balance.

● ● ●

Melanin: The dark, brown pigment found in the skin, eyes, and hair that helps absorb the rays of the sun, protecting the cells from sun damage.

Melanocytes: The skin cells that produce melanin.

Psoriasis: A skin condition characterized by scaly, itchy, dry patches that are white, red, or silver in color. It is a reaction produced by the immune system.

Rosacea: A skin condition characterized by red blotches, often with visible capillaries or small, pus-filled red bumps.

Sebaceous glands: The oil-producing glands found in the dermis that release sebum.

Sebum: An oily substance produced by the sebaceous glands that helps prevent your skin from drying out. Sebum escapes to the surface of the skin via the pores/hair follicles.

Stratum corneum: The very outermost layer of the skin that is made up of dead skin cells.

Subcutaneous tissue: The innermost layer of the skin, also called the hypodermis. It is made up of fat and large blood vessels and helps regulate body temperature.

BIBLIOGRAPHY

ONE: Up Close and Personal

American Academy of Dermatology. "The Layers of Your Skin." Accessed May 15, 2019. https://www.aad.org/public/kids/skin/the-layers-of-your-skin.

Howard, Diana, and the International Dermal Institute. "Structural Changes Associated with Aging Skin." Accessed May 6, 2019. http://www.dermalinstitute.com/us/library/11_article_Structural_Changes_AssociatAs_with_Aging_Skin.html.

TWO: Your Nutrition Routine

Bowe, W. P., and A. R. Shalita. "Effective Over-the-Counter Acne Treatments." *Seminars in Cutaneous Medicine and Surgery* 27, no. 3 (September 2008): 170–76.

Chainy, G. B., S. K. Manna, M. M. Chaturvedi, and B. B. Aggarwal. "Anethole Blocks Both Early and Late Cellular Responses Transduced by Tumor Necrosis Factor." *Oncogene* 19, no. 25 (June 8, 2000): 2943–50.

Cosgrove, Maeve, Oscar H. Franco, Stewart P. Granger, Peter G. Murray, and Andrew E. Mayes. "Dietary Nutrient Intakes and Skin-Aging Appearance Among Middle-Aged American Women." *American Journal of Clinical Nutrition* 86, no. 4 (October 2007): 1225–31.

Herman, Anna. "Caffeine's Mechanisms of Action and Its Cosmetic Use." *Skin Pharmacology and Physiology* 26, no. 1 (2013): 8–14.

Kim, J., Y. Ko, Y. K. Park, N. I. Kim, W. K. Ha, and Y. Cho. "Dietary Effect of Lactoferrin-Enriched Fermented Milk on Skin Surface Lipid and Clinical Improvement of Acne Vulgaris." *Nutrition* 26, no. 9 (September 2010): 902–9.

Li, Suyun, Eunyoung Cho, Aaron M. Drucker, Abrar A. Qureshi, and Wen-Qing Li. "Alcohol Intake and Risk of Rosacea in US Women." *Journal of the American Academy of Dermatology* 76, no. 6 (June 2017): 1061–67.

Li, Suyun, Michael L. Chen, Aaron M. Drucker, Eunyoung Cho, Hao Geng, Abrar A. Qureshi, and Wen-Qing Li. "Association of Caffeine Intake and Caffeinated Coffee Consumption with Risk of Incident Rosacea in Women." *JAMA Dermatology* 154, no. 12 (2018): 1394–1400.

Loftfield, Erikka. "Coffee May Be Associated with a Lower Risk of Malignant Melanoma." *JNCI: Journal of the National Cancer Institute* 107, no. 2 (February 2015).

Mahmassani, Hiya A., Esther E. Avendano, Gowri Raman, and Elizabeth J. Johnson. "Avocado Consumption and Risk Factors for Heart Disease: A Systematic Review and Meta-Analysis." *American Journal of Clinical Nutrition* 107, no. 4 (April 2018): 523–36.

Marchetti, F., R. Capizzi, and A. Tulli. "Efficacy of Regulators of Intestinal Bacterial Flora in the Therapy of Acne Vulgaris." *Clinical Therapeutics* 122, no. 5 (September 15, 1987): 339–43.

Melnik, B. C. "Linking Diet to Acne Metabolomics, Inflammation, and Comedogenesis: An Update." *Clinical Cosmetic and Investigative Dermatology* 8 (July 15, 2015): 371–88.

Rostan, E. F., H. V. DeBuys, D. L. Madey, and S. R. Pinnell. "Evidence Supporting Zinc as an Important Antioxidant for Skin." *International Journal of Dermatology* 41, no. 9 (September 2002): 606–11.

Williams, S., N. Krueger, M. Davids, D. Kraus, and M. Kerscher. "Effect of Fluid Intake on Skin Physiology." *International Journal of Cosmetic Science* 29, no. 2 (April 2007): 131–38.

THREE: Your Skincare Routine

Lourenco, E. A. J., L. Shaw, H. Pratt, G. L. Duffy, G. Czanner, Y. Zheng, K. J. Hammill, and A. G. McCormick. "Application of SPF Moisturizers Is Inferior to Sunscreens in Coverage of Facial and Eyelid Regions." *PLoS One* 14, no. 4 (April 3, 2019).

Qingsu, Xia, Jun J. Yin, Wayne G. Wamer, Shu-Hui Cherng, Mary D. Boudreau, Paul C. Howard, Hongtao Yu, and Peter P. Fu. "Photoirradiation of Retinyl Palmitate in Ethanol with Ultraviolet Light—Formation of Photodecomposition Products, Reactive Oxygen Species, and Lipid Peroxides." *International Journal of Environmental Research and Public Health* 3, no. 2 (June 30, 2006): 185–90.

Sundaram, Hema. "Role of Physiologically Balanced Growth Factors in Skin Rejuvenation." *Journal of Drugs in Dermatology* 8, no. 5 (May 2009).

Trehean, Sonia, Bozena Michniak-Kohn, and Kavita Beri. "Plant Stem Cells in Cosmetics: Current Trends and Future Directions." *Future Science OA* 3, no. 4 (November 2017).

FOUR: Your Self-Care Routine

Epel, Elissa, Jennifer Daubenmier, Judith T. Moskowitz, Susan Folkman, and Elizabeth Blackburn. "Can Meditation Slow Rate of Cellular Aging? Cognitive Stress, Mindfulness, and Telomeres." *Annals of the New York Academy of Sciences* 1172 (August 2009): 34–53.

Faraut, B., K. Z. Boudjeltia, L. Vanhamme, and M. Kerkhofs. "Immune, Inflammatory and Cardiovascular Consequences of Sleep Restriction and Recovery." *Sleep Medicine Reviews* 16, no. 2 (April 2012): 137–49.

Gomez-Cabrera, Mari-Carmen, Elena Domenech, and Jose Viña. "Moderate Exercise Is an Antioxidant: Upregulation of Antioxidant Genes by Training." *Free Radical Biology and Medicine* 44, no. 2 (January 15, 2008): 126–31.

London School of Hygiene and Tropical Medicine. "Contamination of UK Mobile Phones and Hands Revealed." October 14, 2011. https://www.lshtm.ac.uk/newsevents/news/2011/mobilephones.html.

Safdar, Adeel, Jacqueline M. Bourgeois, Daniel I. Ogborn, Jonathan P. Little, Bart P. Hettinga, Mahmood Akhtar, James E. Thompson, et al. "Endurance Exercise Rescues Progeroid Aging and Induces Systemic Mitochondrial Rejuvenation in MTDNA Mutator Mice." *PNAS* 108, no. 10 (March 8, 2011): 4135–40.

INDEX

stem cells, *see* EGFs (epidermal growth factors)

stratum corneum, 6, 11, 108, 133, 134–35, 185, 251

stress management, 137–41

subcutaneous tissue (hypodermis), xvii, 6, 9, 15, 251

sugar, 22, 26, 47–48, 53–56, 76, 138, 197–207, 222–23

"sugar face," 55

sun damage, 28, 36, 92–96, 123–24, 162–63, 210–11, 222, 245, 248

sunscreen:
    chemical sunscreens and, 94–95, 208
    mineral-based sunscreen, 95–96
    in moisturizers, 87–88
    product recommendations and, 96
    skincare routine and, 92–96

Supernova Serum, 124

T

technology, in skincare field, 162–67, 171, 187
    see also specialty treatments

"Time Machine, The" light bed, 166

time-targeted routines, 217–26
    one-day, 225–26
    one-month, 221–23
    one-week, 223–25
    six-month, 218–21

toners, 63, 125–26, 200–202

towels, 68, 99, 191, 197, 202

turmeric, 15, 36–37

Twilight Masks, 105–6

V

Vitamin B$_2$, 25

Vitamin B$_3$, 91

Vitamin C, 23–25, 52, 90, 222

Vitamin C Face Wash, 70, 73, 212

Vitamin D, 24

Vitamin E, 24, 28, 32, 66, 90–91, 118, 211

Vitamin K, 25, 78, 198

vitamins, 21, 24–25, 39, 51–52, 235

W

water, 33–36, 61, 139
    see also dehydration

wrinkles:
    causes of, 11, 92, 103, 139, 150
    elimination of, 19, 80, 90, 103, 108, 114, 120–23, 162, 174, 228
    mask recipes for, 239, 243, 248
    prevention of, 27, 31–38, 143–46
    troubleshooting, 211–12

Y

Yoon, Alicia, 74
    see also Peach & Lily

Z

Zinc, 25, 31, 78, 114, 197, 201, 211

JOANNA VARGAS is a recognized skin care expert and the founder of an eponymous skin care collection. With salons in New York City and Los Angeles, her commitment to plant-based ingredients, her passion for science, and her nature-meets-technology approach has made her one of the most sought-out aestheticians and experts in the beauty industry today.

Bringing her background in photography and a BA in women's studies into the beauty industry, Joanna navigated her way through her early days as a facialist in New York City. Joanna first fell in love with natural skin care products while practicing aesthetics at a day spa and later worked for a celebrity dermatologist, where she learned extensively about anti-aging treatments and the most efficacious ingredients and formulas available. Today, Julianne Moore, Rachel Brosnahan, Mindy Kaling, Sofia Coppola, and Jake Gyllenhaal are just a few famous faces who look to Joanna for radiant skin.

Joanna lives in New Jersey with her husband and two children.

HarperCollins books may be purchased for educational, business, or sales promotional use. For information, please email the Special Markets Department at SPsales@harpercollins.com.

FIRST EDITION

Designed by Bonni Leon-Berman

Library of Congress Cataloging-in-Publication Data has been applied for.

ISBN 978-0-06-290913-8

20 21 22 23 24   LSC   10 9 8 7 6 5 4 3 2 1